THE
EVERYTHING®
GUIDE TO
THE CARB CYCLING DIET

Dear Reader,

When I began my fitness journey, I was a year into college and had no idea how I should be eating. I played sports all through high school, but once that ended, my bad eating habits caught up to me, and I knew it was time to try to lose some weight.

This was about eight years ago. When I first started, I tried every diet under the sun—Paleo, Intermittent Fasting, counting calories, just clean eating, bodybuilder-style diets, you name it. I've found that carbohydrate cycling simply made the most sense, in terms of results and health benefits. I have seen great results, and find it very easy to stick to.

I've also helped many clients all over the world who want to lose some weight, and by far, they've found carb cycling the most sustainable and easy-to-follow plan. I'm confident that if you read this book and implement the diet in your own life, you'll find that you can finally obtain the body you've always wanted, without giving up your favorite foods or being miserable.

Best of luck on your road to a leaner body, and always remember to take time to enjoy the journey.

Matt Dustin, CSCS, Pn1

Welcome to the EVERYTHING® Series!

These handy, accessible books give you all you need to tackle a difficult project, gain a new hobby, comprehend a fascinating topic, prepare for an exam, or even brush up on something you learned back in school but have since forgotten.

You can choose to read an Everything® book from cover to cover or just pick out the information you want from our four useful boxes: e-questions, e-facts, e-alerts, and e-ssentials.

We give you everything you need to know on the subject, but throw in a lot of fun stuff along the way, too.

We now have more than 400 Everything® books in print, spanning such wide-ranging categories as weddings, pregnancy, cooking, music instruction, foreign language, crafts, pets, New Age, and so much more. When you're done reading them all, you can finally say you know Everything®!

QUESTION

Answers to
common questions

FACT

Important snippets
of information

ALERT

Urgent
warnings

ESSENTIAL

Quick
handy tips

PUBLISHER Karen Cooper

MANAGING EDITOR, EVERYTHING® SERIES Lisa Laing

COPY CHIEF Casey Ebert

ASSISTANT PRODUCTION EDITOR Jo-Anne Duhamel

ACQUISITIONS EDITOR Hillary Thompson

SENIOR DEVELOPMENT EDITOR Brett Palana-Shanahan

EVERYTHING® SERIES COVER DESIGNER Erin Alexander

Visit the entire Everything® series at *www.everything.com*

THE
EVERYTHING®
GUIDE TO THE CARB CYCLING DIET

An effective diet plan to lose weight
and boost your metabolism

Matt Dustin, CSCS, Pn1

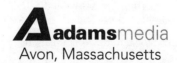

Avon, Massachusetts

This book is dedicated to all of you readers who have struggled to reach your dream body. I've been there, and I sincerely hope this book helps you reach your goals.

An Everything® Series Book.
Everything® and everything.com® are registered trademarks of F+W Media, Inc.

Published by
Adams Media, a division of F+W Media, Inc.
57 Littlefield Street, Avon, MA 02322. U.S.A.
www.adamsmedia.com

Contains material adapted from *The Everything® DASH Diet Cookbook* by Christy Ellingsworth and Murdoc Khaleghi, copyright © 2012 by F+W Media, Inc., ISBN 10: 1-4405-4353-4, ISBN 13: 978-1-4405-4353-1; *The Everything® Eating Clean Cookbook* by Britt Brandon, copyright © 2012 by F+W Media, Inc., ISBN 10: 1-4405-2999-X, ISBN 13: 978-1-4405-2999-3; *The Everything® Whole Foods Cookbook* by Rachel Rappaport, copyright © 2012 by F+W Media, Inc., ISBN 10: 1-4405-3168-4, ISBN 13: 978-1-4405-3168-2; *The Everything® Eating Clean Cookbook for Vegetarians* by Britt Brandon, copyright © 2013 by F+W Media, Inc., ISBN 10: 1-4405-5140-5, ISBN 13: 978-1-4405-5140-6; *The Everything® Low-Glycemic Cookbook* by Carrie S. Forbes, copyright © 2014 by F+W Media, Inc., ISBN 10: 1-4405-7086-8, ISBN 13: 978-1-4405-7086-5.

ISBN 10: 1-4405-9516-X
ISBN 13: 978-1-4405-9516-5
eISBN 10: 1-4405-9517-8
eISBN 13: 978-1-4405-9517-2

Printed in the United States of America.

10   9   8   7   6   5   4   3   2   1

Library of Congress Cataloging-in-Publication Data
Dustin, Matt, author.
The everything guide to the carb cycling diet : an effective diet plan
  to lose weight and boost your metabolism / Matt Dustin, CSCS, Pn1.
Avon, Massachusetts : Adams Media, [2016] | Series:
  Everything;
Includes index.
LCCN 2015045526 | ISBN 9781440595165 (pb) | ISBN
  144059516X (pb) | ISBN 9781440595172 (ebook) | ISBN 1440595178
  (ebook)
LCSH: Low-carbohydrate diet. | BASIC: HEALTH & FITNESS / Diets. |
  COOKING / Health & Healing / Low Carbohydrate.
LCC RM237.73 .D87 2016 | DDC 641.5/6383--dc23
LC record available at *http://lccn.loc.gov/2015045526*

The information in this book should not be used for diagnosing or treating any health problem. Not all diet and exercise plans suit everyone. You should always consult a trained medical professional before starting a diet, taking any form of medication, or embarking on any fitness or weight-training program. The author and publisher disclaim any liability arising directly or indirectly from the use of this book.

Many of the designations used by manufacturers and sellers to distinguish their products are claimed as trademarks. Where those designations appear in this book and F+W Media, Inc. was aware of a trademark claim, the designations have been printed with initial capital letters.

Cover image © StockFood/Sven Benjamins.

This book is available at quantity discounts for bulk purchases.
For information, please call 1-800-289-0963.

Contents

Introduction 11

1   **What Is Carb Cycling?** 13

What Are Macronutrients? 14

Identifying Carbohydrates, Proteins, and Fats. 16

Fiber's Role in Counting Carbs 19

What Carb Cycling Is Not. 20

The Basics: High-Carb Days and Low-Carb Days 21

How the Body Loses Fat. 22

Counting Calories with Carb Cycling 23

2   **The Benefits of Cycling Your
Carbohydrate Intake** 25

How Carbohydrates Impact Your Body 26

Problems with High Carbohydrate Intake 27

Stabilizing Blood Sugar and Losing Fat 28

Boosting Mental Clarity, Focus, and Energy 29

Outsmarting Hunger and Staying on Track 30

Improving Your Hormonal Profile. 31

Building a Caloric Deficit for Fat Loss 31

Enjoying the Foods You Like—in Moderation! 34

3 How to Get Started 35

Scheduling High-Carb and Low-Carb Days 36

Determining Your Intake Levels 37

Meal Planning: Your Key to Success 41

Food Shopping and Preparation 42

Good and Bad Nutrient Combos 43

Scheduling "Cheat" Meals 43

Tips and Tricks to Maximize Your Results 44

4 Advanced Carb Cycling Strategies 47

Adding Exercise 48

Endurance Training versus Strength Training 49

Cycling Carbs Around Your Workouts 54

Breaking Through Fat-Loss Plateaus 55

5 The Maintenance Phase 59

Do You Need to Carb Cycle Forever? 60

Transitioning to a "Normal" Eating Style 61

The Importance of Reverse Dieting 61

Carb Cycling for Maintenance and for Life 63

Instinctive Eating versus Carb Cycling 64

Working in High-Carb Days Without Gaining Fat 65

How to Use the Resources in This Book 66

6 Breakfast 69

7 Lunch 85

8 Dinner: Beef, Pork, and Poultry 101

9 Dinner: Fish and Shellfish 117

10 Vegetarian Mains, Sides, and Salads 127

11 Vegan Mains, Sides, and Salads 141

12 Pasta 157

13 Soups 169

14 Sauces, Dressings, and Rubs 181

15 Sides 191

16 Snacks 207

17 Holidays 217

18 Drinks 239

19 Desserts 249

Appendix A:
Sample Menu Plan for High-Carb and
Low-Carb Days 261

Appendix B:
Best Food Sources for Each
Macronutrient Group 265

Appendix C:
FAQ. 269

Appendix D:
Additional Resources 273

Standard U.S./Metric Measurement
Conversions 275

Index. 277

Acknowledgments

First of all, I'd like to thank Hillary Thompson, and everyone at Adams Media, for helping me through the process of publishing my first book. It's been a wonderful experience, and I've learned a lot along the way. I'd also like to thank all of the various editors who have been kind enough to give me a shot and publish my work over the last few years; I wouldn't be where I am today without those opportunities.

Thanks to the awesome folks at Influx Cafe here in San Diego for supplying the best coffee around and keeping me fueled as I wrote this. Lastly, a huge thank you to all the clients I've had the honor of working with over the last five years—I've learned so much from you all, and wouldn't be the trainer and coach I am today without you.

Introduction

IN THE WORLD OF dieting, there are countless options and plans for you to follow. Many are based on extreme restrictions, eliminating one food group or another. Some are based around timing of meals, counting calories or points, or just eating "clean" foods. It can be very confusing, and with so many options, it's hard to know which is the best. When you consider the number of options and the fact that most of them use very dramatic before and after stories and pictures in their marketing, you might be tempted to just give up all together.

The truth is, the best diet is the one you can stick to. Any plan that has you eating less food than you need will help you lose fat. The difference is that some plans make this easy and fun, and some make it downright miserable. The last thing you want to hear is that you can't eat a certain food, because as soon as something is forbidden, chances are you'll crave it even more.

With that being said, carbohydrate cycling is one of the easiest methods you can use to remove unwanted body fat. It takes a bit of planning, but the execution is very easy and painless. There are no restrictions, as any food you enjoy can be made to fit in the plan. It's intuitive, and makes sense once you learn a little bit about how your body processes and uses food. In addition to helping you lose fat, carbohydrate cycling can have a whole host of other benefits as well, which is something that not all diet plans can say.

This book will take you through the entire process, giving you all the tools you'll need to begin your journey and actually see sustainable results. You'll learn what carb cycling is and what it isn't. You'll learn about macronutrients, how your body uses the food you eat, and the impact exercise has on your body. After reading, you'll know how to plan for social events, vacations, or any other time you want to eat a lot of your favorite foods, without undoing all of your progress. Finally, this book will show you exactly how to figure out how much food you should be eating and how to set up a carb cycling plan that suits your life.

By the end of the book, you will know how to start your program and manipulate it as you go, and you'll have a whole bunch of recipes to get you started. It takes time and results won't happen overnight, but with a little patience and some hard work, you'll be able to reduce your body fat levels and finally earn your dream body.

Perhaps most importantly, this book will also teach you what to do after you have reached your initial goals on the diet. Most books teach you how to eat and work out to reach your goal, and end with the assumption that you'll get your dream body. Even if you do reach your goals, what comes after is just as important, as returning immediately to your old habits is a surefire way to gain all the weight back. This plan will show how to transition from dieting mode to a maintenance mode that you can easily maintain for life.

CHAPTER 1

What Is Carb Cycling?

Carb cycling is a dietary approach that allows you to optimize your body composition by losing fat and building lean muscle, without the stress of extreme food limitations or calorie counting. By strategically manipulating the amount of carbohydrates you consume on a daily basis, it is easy to set up a fat-burning environment in your body, one that can be maintained easily and for long periods of time.

What Are Macronutrients?

Before anything can be discussed about carb cycling, it's important to first define what exactly a carbohydrate is. Your body relies on food to live, and uses the calories consumed through food to perform all the functions of daily living. All calories come from macronutrients, which are carbohydrates, proteins, and fats. A calorie is simply a unit of measurement used to describe the amount of energy gained from consuming a certain food.

ESSENTIAL

Macronutrients are proteins, carbs, and fat. You can remember this because macro means large. Micronutrients, on the other hand, while essential, don't have any calories. Micronutrients would include vitamins, minerals, antioxidants, and other things found in food that don't have any calories.

Where Do Calories Come From?

When caloric values from food are calculated for labeling purposes, it is the macronutrients that are being measured. A gram of carbohydrate has 4 calories, a gram of protein has 4 calories, and a gram of fat has 9 calories. Vitamins and minerals, also called micronutrients, are essential to optimum functioning of the human body, but do not provide any caloric value. So when you look at a label, all that gets factored into the total calories are the protein, carb, and fat totals. These are listed in grams, while other nutrients may be listed in other measurements, or even percentages of your daily recommended intake.

ESSENTIAL

You may be curious about how alcohol fits in. While it has both benefits and negative effects, speaking strictly in terms of calories, alcohol is an oddity. It has 7 calories per gram, more than protein and carbs but less than fat. However, it doesn't provide any nutrients, so it is purely empty calories. Wine, beer, and sugary mixed drinks will usually have carbohydrates as well, but pure liquor only has alcohol calories.

A healthy diet will consist of a proper balance of all three macronutrients, as all are essential for optimal living. You may be able to get by with low intake of one, but it's generally not going to have you feel your best. For example, you can go very long periods of time without any carbohydrate intake, as long as protein and fat intake are adequate, but your energy levels and recovery from physical activity will suffer. If you go low-fat for long periods of time, you can suffer from all sorts of negative hormonal effects, such as decreased testosterone in both men and women, and lowered estrogen in women. Low testosterone and estrogen can lead to a decrease in sex drive, lower energy, and a higher body fat to lean mass ratio.

What Do the Macros Do?

Proteins are used to rebuild many different cells in the body, and benefit skin, hair, fingernails, muscle growth, and many other functions. You may have heard that you need protein to build muscle, and this is true, which makes it easy to remember that you need protein to repair and build just about anything in your body. Proteins are the building blocks of the body.

Fats are generally slower to digest, provide a satiating, or hunger-blunting, effect, and are necessary for optimal hormonal profiles. There are a lot of misconceptions about fat, and many diets suggest eating as little fat as possible, but this is not smart or healthy. Sure, some types of fats are better than others, but you need fat to live, and the right fats are very beneficial to your body. During times of restricted carbohydrate intake, fat becomes even more important to supply energy.

QUESTION

Doesn't fat make you fat?
No. This is a very common belief, because they share the same name, but this is not true. Dietary fat, which you eat in your food, is essential for your body in certain amounts. Adipose tissue, or body fat, is simply stored calories. While eating high-fat foods *can* make you fat, fats consumed in the correct amounts will not cause you to become fat.

Carbohydrates are an interesting macronutrient. While not technically necessary to survive—as your body can break down protein and convert it into a form of glucose, which is what carbohydrates are made of—they provide a fast-digesting, readily available energy source. Once broken down into glucose, they elevate blood sugar levels and provide energy to the body, and are used during higher-intensity activities, such as exercise, sports, or physical jobs.

FACT

Some people will tell you that carbohydrates are essential to stay alive, since your brain needs glucose to function. However, through a cool little process called gluconeogenesis, or the conversion of protein to carbs, your body can actually make glucose without carbs. It takes a while, and it's not ideal, but it can be done.

In terms of body composition, no single macronutrient is the key to reaching your goal, and no macronutrient alone is responsible for fat. You can consume any food in excess and gain fat. To function at optimal levels, you should eat protein, carbs, and fat in the proper amounts, and avoid completely eliminating any one of those nutrients.

Identifying Carbohydrates, Proteins, and Fats

Now that the macronutrients have been defined, it's important to be able to identify what types of foods each comes from. You may know that you need to eat high-protein foods, but you also need to know what those foods are. Many whole food sources will predominantly be one macronutrient or the other, with some protein sources containing fat as well. With highly processed foods, it is not so easy to know what is what, so it's important to check the nutrition label as you shop and plan for your meals.

Where Do Macros Come From?

Carbohydrates are found in starchy food sources, fruits, and vegetables. Common sources include potatoes, rice, and high-sugar fruits such as bananas, grapes, and mangos. To a lesser extent, carbohydrates are also found in vegetables, although often in much lower quantities. The highest carbohydrate levels are found in processed sugary food, such as cereal, bread, rice, pasta, crackers, dried fruit, and soft drinks.

Protein is something to pay special attention to. A complete protein is made up of twenty different amino acids, all of which have varying roles in the body. The more types of amino acids a protein contains, the more complete it is considered. Most of the tissue in your body is composed of amino acids, which are the building blocks of protein and your body, so it's important to get adequate amounts of all twenty amino acids.

Not all food sources contain all twenty of these amino acids, so the more aminos a protein has, the more "complete" it is considered. Among those amino acids are essential amino acids, which are the amino acids your body needs, but cannot produce itself. You must get these essential amino acids by consuming protein sources. The best sources of complete protein are eggs, chicken, fish, beef, pork, and dairy products. While a few plant sources such as beans and nuts may contain trace amounts of protein, they often don't have all twenty amino acids. If you follow a vegetarian diet, you may have to combine several plant sources together to obtain all twenty amino acids, since you won't be getting them from meat sources.

ESSENTIAL

You may have heard all about quinoa, as it is a very trendy healthy food option. While quinoa is not a high-protein food, it does have a wide variety of amino acids in it, and as far as plants go, is a very good source of complete protein. If you're looking to add non-meat protein to your diet, quinoa is a great option.

Fats are most commonly found in nuts, avocados, oils, and high-fat protein sources, such as salmon, egg yolks, certain cuts of red meat, fattier cuts of pork, and dairy products such as butter and cheese. Many processed foods you see at the store will also be very high in fat. As previously mentioned, fat is dense in calories, so high-fat foods will have significantly higher calorie counts. Always remember that while fat is essential for living, a gram of fat will have over twice the calories of a gram of protein or carbohydrate, so you don't want to consume unlimited amounts of fat.

As you begin considering what sorts of foods you want to keep in the house, here is a list of the best food sources for each macronutrient. When consumed on a regular basis, these foods supply plenty of good micronutrients and antioxidants, and provide a variety of nutrients to your body. Other foods are acceptable, of course, but the ones listed here will provide healthy, nutritious sources for your macronutrients, and should be the foundation of most of your meals.

FACT

Antioxidants help protect the body from free radicals, which can damage the healthy cells in your body. Free radicals can be created by your body's regular function, stressful situations, or by exposure to environmental toxins, such as pollution, smoke, and herbicides. Antioxidants neutralize the threat of the free radicals by affecting their electrical charge, preventing them from damaging other cells.

BEST PROTEIN SOURCES:

- Boneless, skinless chicken breast
- Whole eggs/egg whites
- Lean turkey breast or ground turkey
- Low-fat fish
- Low-fat red meat
- Low-fat cottage cheese

BEST CARBOHYDRATE SOURCES:

- Potatoes (any color)
- Rice
- Fruits and vegetables, in a variety of colors
- Oats

BEST FAT SOURCES:

- Nuts
- Avocados
- Coconut oil
- High-fat cuts of red meat
- High-fat fish
- Whole eggs

ESSENTIAL

You may have heard that fish is a good source of healthy fats, and this is mostly true. Fish tends to be higher in omega-3 fatty acids, which are very good for your body. However, there is a difference in fat levels in various fish. Typically, white fish such as tilapia, cod, and flounder are low in fat. Darker fish, such as salmon, mackerel, or tuna, will often have higher fat content. The lower-fat fish will still have beneficial omega-3s, just less of them, and less total fat.

Fiber's Role in Counting Carbs

It is also necessary to define fiber, as many different brands and companies include it in different ways. Fiber is a part of certain carbohydrates that generally consists of much denser material. Your body has a harder time digesting fiber, so if you consume higher amounts of fiber, you will most likely notice that you stay full longer. In terms of health benefits, fiber can improve digestion, blood sugar levels, frequency of bowel movements, and is generally very helpful to include in your diet.

Because fiber is so dense and hard to digest, many labeling or diet systems remove fiber from the total carbohydrate count. So, a food with 20 grams of carbohydrate and 5 grams of fiber may list "15 net carbs" on the label, because the 5 grams of fiber don't digest as quickly as starchy carbs.

However, it is still important to look at total carbs, as fiber doesn't cancel them out, contrary to what some labels would have you believe. Adding fiber powder to ice cream, for example, would not nullify the effects of the high sugar levels found in the ice cream. If this worked, you could simply carry around a fiber supplement and consume it with all your carbs to cancel them out, which unfortunately would not work well. You always have to look at the total carbohydrates.

FACT

If you've ever read about carbohydrates, you may be familiar with the glycemic index. The glycemic index is a measure of how fast carbohydrates raise blood sugar levels. Highly processed carbs have a high glycemic index, as they spike your blood sugar quickly. Carbs high in fiber have a much lower number on the glycemic index, which is why they are often recommended—you want stable blood sugar levels, not spikes up and down all day.

Fibrous food sources include green leafy vegetables, some fruits, and whole-grain carbohydrate sources such as oatmeal. It is also possible to add fiber supplements to a diet if the diet does not provide adequate fiber; however, you should always consult a healthcare professional before taking any dietary supplements. When following the plans in this book, always count total carbohydrates; don't subtract fiber from the total.

What Carb Cycling Is Not

There are many popular diets out there, and quite a few are based around the idea that carbs make you fat, and thus must be eliminated. It doesn't matter if you eat unlimited amounts of fat and protein, according to these diets, because carbs are the true evil. This is not true.

Carbohydrate cycling is simply a way of eating that allows you to have varying carb intakes on different days of the week. It is not an elimination diet, where carbs are banned in all forms indefinitely. It is also not a low-fat diet—on low-carb days, fat may actually be quite high to reach the necessary caloric intake level. Carb levels fluctuate when using cycling, versus an all-or-nothing approach that has been made popular by so many other diets.

The Basics: High-Carb Days and Low-Carb Days

The most basic form of carb cycling is to have two levels of carbohydrate intake: high and low. Other methods will be detailed later on, with varying daily levels of carbohydrate intake, but for now only high and low days will be discussed.

High-Carb Days

On higher-carb days, carb sources will include rice, pasta, fruit, and potatoes—traditional starchy carbohydrate sources. High-carb days should fall on days with high physical activity. If physical activity is not a normal routine, then high-carb days should be set around personal preference, such as on the weekends to allow for social indulgences.

On higher-carb days, protein intake should stay roughly the same, with an emphasis on lower-fat sources. Since carb intake is higher, total calories will also increase, so to offset this, total fat should be lowered. Calories must be controlled for weight loss to happen, so people who use carb cycling to lose fat should remember to always keep total calories roughly the same each day.

ALERT

A common misconception in the world of dieting is that if carbs are kept very low, you can eat as much "other" food as you want without consequence. Always watch the fat content in your food, as fat has more than twice as many calories as carbs, gram for gram. It's very possible to be on a low-carb diet and gain body fat if total food intake is too high.

Low-Carb Days

On low-carb days, carb intake should be set very low. Most meals should come from proteins and vegetables, with the daily carb intake being limited to the trace carbs in vegetables and maybe one serving of fruit. It's important to avoid drinking anything with excessive amounts of carbs, as this can defeat the purpose of a low-carb day. Just as with the high-carb day, fat will be adjusted. On this type of day, however, fat intake should increase, since carbs are decreased.

How the Body Loses Fat

To understand why this works, and why some of the rules that will be laid out are necessary, it's important to first have a general understanding of how fat loss and gain occur in the body. There are so many rumors about fat loss that just aren't true. Fat doesn't just melt away, or turn into muscle, and your body probably won't store pounds of fat off of one big meal.

First, body fat is simply stored energy. As mentioned earlier, food is measured in calories, a unit of measurement to describe the amount of energy gained from that food. All daily activities of living, plus any and all physical activity, use these calories. If you are moving around all day, you'll burn more calories than if you sat down all day. So, if a diet provides more calories than are needed, your body will look to store the excess as energy in muscle, or as adipose tissue, which is the actual fat on the body.

Total Food Intake Is What Matters

When you are consistently in a caloric excess, weight will be gained, as you are eating more calories than your body can use. If someone is looking to add muscle and is following a proper workout program, this may be desired. However, for fat loss, there must be a caloric deficit—that is, eating fewer calories than you burn.

The first law of thermodynamics applies here: energy cannot be created or destroyed, only transformed. If your body uses more calories than it takes in, it has to get the energy from somewhere, and stored fat is a perfect place. If you eat too many calories, you'll gain body fat. This is why a caloric deficit causes fat loss, and absolutely must be in place for fat loss to occur.

Without this caloric deficit, you cannot reduce body fat. There are no secret workouts, pills, magic foods, or anything else that can get around this rule. Some diets will try to severely limit fat or carbohydrate intake. The reason this is effective is because by removing those food groups, a caloric deficit is created. However, there is nothing inherently evil about any food group; all that matters in the end is maintaining a caloric deficit.

Once your body reaches the point where energy output is greater than intake, it will start to metabolize, or break down and use, body fat. The fat cells are transported to the cells of our bodies that will break them down for energy, or "burn" them. So, the body breaks down fat and transports it to be used for energy, and this energy is then used for calorie-burning activities, with the waste being removed through sweat, urine, and exhaling of breath.

FACT

Many people believe that sweating profusely during a workout means you are losing fat. If you notice that you are several pounds lighter after a workout, it's possible some of that was fat, but odds are that most of that weight was water lost through sweating, not actual fat loss. Always remember to rehydrate yourself and drink plenty of fluids after any activity where you are heavily sweating.

Counting Calories with Carb Cycling

You know that you must control total calories to lose body fat. However, this doesn't necessarily mean you need to count them each day. While this may be a smart move in many cases, depending on your level of discipline, you may be able to see great results without counting calories on a regular basis.

Just by the nature of restricting carbs on certain days, odds are you are creating a sufficient caloric deficit, at least if you have a decent amount of fat to lose. If your food choices stay generally the same, with lowered carbs on certain days, you shouldn't have too much trouble losing fat, at least initially.

However, if you find yourself eating foods you wouldn't normally eat, especially high-fat foods, you may find yourself in trouble. There is nothing wrong with eating high-fat foods in moderation, so long as you still make sure you aren't overshooting your total daily calorie goal. For example, if your protein sources stay the same, and you add a few extra eggs, or an avocado, on your low-carb day, you'll probably be okay. However, if you start eating eggs, bacon, steak, handfuls of nuts all day—you may be eating too much fat.

Later on in this book you'll learn how to figure out how many calories you should be eating to maintain or lose weight, but for now, just know that it isn't necessary to count calories if you have the self-control to avoid high-fat foods on your low-carb days. Start without counting. Mindfully follow the plans that will come later in the book, and see what happens. If you find you aren't seeing the results you want, you may have to start counting calories for a while.

CHAPTER 2

The Benefits of Cycling Your Carbohydrate Intake

There are many benefits of cycling your carbohydrate intake beyond merely improving your rate of fat loss. From helping control your hunger and energy levels to improving mental focus and even improving your hormonal profile, carbohydrate cycling can do a lot of great things for your body. It's important to first understand what actually happens when you eat carbohydrates, in terms of digestion and the subsequent effects, and then you can fully understand and implement the benefits of cycling.

How Carbohydrates Impact Your Body

You already know what carbohydrates are and where they come from. Now it's time to understand what happens to them once they are consumed. The process begins with digestion. During the digestion phase, your body works to break down the carbohydrates into single molecules of glucose. Depending on the type of carbohydrate, this breakdown may be fast or slow. Simple carbohydrates will be digested more quickly than complex carbohydrates, as they can be broken down faster, which is an important point to remember moving forward.

ESSENTIAL

Glucose is the substance that will be mentioned the most frequently here, as it is the body's preferred source of energy. It is most commonly found in grains, potatoes, rice, and other starchy foods. However, a very similar molecule called fructose, found mainly in fruit, has a similar effect on blood sugar, and is also very quickly digested. So while fruit doesn't have glucose, it does break down into fructose, which is nearly the same thing.

As part of the digestion process, the glucose is next absorbed into the bloodstream, where it can be carried around to places that need it, or it could be stored in adipose tissue (body fat cells) for later use. Eating a large portion of carbohydrates will elevate your blood sugar levels, with simple carbohydrates resulting in a fast increase and complex carbohydrates resulting in a slower, more stable increase.

ALERT

Blood sugar is important to monitor. While it's not necessarily bad to have high blood sugar short-term, chronically high blood sugar can increase one's risk of becoming pre-diabetic, or developing diabetes later in life. Ideally, blood sugar should be kept as stable as possible. If it's too low, you'll feel tired and can get dizzy or lightheaded, and if it gets too high too quickly, you'll experience an energy rush followed by a sharp crash, which can make you feel tired and moody.

Problems with High Carbohydrate Intake

In response to blood sugar being elevated, your body will seek to process the glucose as quickly as possible. When your body senses an elevation in blood sugar, it signals the pancreas to release insulin, which will help clear the blood of glucose and get it stored properly. Insulin encourages your body to store nutrients that are in the bloodstream, so whether it's glucose from carbohydrates, amino acids from proteins, or fatty acids, your body will look to move these to storage when insulin is released. Nutrients can be stored in muscles or various organs to replenish their stores, but if those stores are full, and the nutrients won't be burned for energy, they will be stored as fat tissue. If you are eating high-sugar foods on a regular basis, your body will have to use more insulin. The more you have to use insulin to lower blood sugar levels, the less effective it becomes, almost like developing a tolerance for caffeine, which becomes less effective with chronic use, requiring more and more to get the desired effect.

When you have chronically elevated blood sugar, your body requires greater amounts of insulin to handle the sugar load, which over time can increase your risk of developing type 2 diabetes, a condition where your body can't produce enough insulin to control your blood sugar, causing your blood sugar levels to rise too high. With type 2 diabetes you lose your insulin sensitivity, meaning you need more and more insulin to do the same amount of work. Eventually your pancreas just can't produce enough insulin to keep up. In type 1 diabetes, which is a condition you are born with, your body simply doesn't produce insulin, so you'll need to inject it on a regular basis or have an insulin pump that automatically keeps insulin in your system at all times.

ESSENTIAL

Carbohydrate cycling can help improve your insulin sensitivity. By utilizing long periods of lowered carbohydrate intake, you can allow your body to reset itself and learn to utilize insulin properly again. Improved insulin sensitivity is just one of the many health benefits of cycling your carbohydrate intake, in addition to helping your body use carbohydrates more efficiently rather than storing them as fat.

It's important to note that much of this negative blood sugar spiking can be negated by choosing complex, high-fiber carbs and spreading them over a period of time. It's still a great idea to cycle your carbohydrate intake on a day-to-day basis, as the glucose will eventually make it to your blood-stream regardless of the source, but high-fiber, complex carbs can reduce the amount of fast blood sugar spikes. The fast spikes and subsequent drops in blood sugar that come from eating simple carbs can cause fatigue, hunger, mood swings, headaches, and other negative effects, so it's best to avoid this as much as possible.

Stabilizing Blood Sugar and Losing Fat

Stabilizing your blood sugar will greatly aid you in your efforts to lose fat. Most of the following information will apply to your higher-carbohydrate days, where you will indeed be taking in carbs throughout the day, but it's useful information to know. If your carbs are highly processed, simple sources, you may suffer blood sugar crashes that come from a high dose of processed carbs, crashes that leave you feeling very cranky and hungry. If you've ever eaten a bag of candy or a doughnut or two, you'll know that it doesn't keep you anywhere near as full as a bowl of oatmeal might, even though the total carbohydrate count might be the same. When trying to diet and exercise self-control, the last thing you need is to feel cranky and hungry from a blood sugar crash. Ultimately, total calories are all that really matter when losing fat, but if you can keep your energy levels, mood, and hunger under control, you'll have a much easier time sticking to a nutrition plan.

QUESTION

Fruits and vegetables have carbohydrates, but aren't they supposed to be healthy?
Fruits and vegetables are an excellent source of a variety of vitamins and minerals, which you need for optimal health, so yes, they are very healthy for you. With vegetables, you'll usually be getting a lot of fiber as well, especially with many types of greens, so you shouldn't worry about those. Fruits, while very healthy, are also full of sugar, so be careful with them if you're worried about blood sugar. It's natural sugar, but sugar nonetheless, and it can cause blood sugar spikes if consumed in large quantities.

As a side effect of trying to control your blood sugar levels, you'll most likely be reducing your calories, and end up speeding up your fat-loss efforts. By stabilizing your blood sugar, you'll improve your mood and reduce your cravings, and this is generally achieved by reducing your simple carbohydrate intake—the two have a synergistic relationship that works very well to help you stay on your plan. You'll eat fewer processed carbs, have better energy and mood throughout the day, and experience fewer hunger cravings caused by blood sugar drops.

Boosting Mental Clarity, Focus, and Energy

Stabilizing blood sugar and reducing the ups and downs associated with carbohydrate intake generally results in better mental functioning as well. This may not seem like a big factor when you are considering starting a diet, but once the negative symptoms start to come out, you'll know exactly why they can make dieting miserable. Steady blood sugar levels will allow you to feel happier and less cranky when dieting, provide you with sustained energy all day, and help you avoid the brain fog you can often feel from restricted carbs and/or fatigue.

Carbohydrates do provide energy for the body, and you will use glucose for many functions of daily living, so it's important to have some in your body. The goal is to have sustained energy all day, however, not big rushes of energy followed by crashes, which can make you want to seek that rush again. If you eat a big, sugary breakfast, such as a bagel and fruit, you'll probably notice a crash later in your workday, when you feel tired, unable to focus, hungry, and moody. You don't want that. If you choose high-fiber, whole-food carb sources, and spread them out throughout the day, you'll most likely feel full longer, feel energized throughout the day, and feel alert and focused.

It's important to note that it may take a little time to adapt to fewer carbohydrates, or a reduction in the sugary ones. If you are used to eating a lot of carbs each day, the first time you try to reduce or eliminate them, you may feel cranky, and feel that your brain is foggy—meaning that it seems harder to focus and process things—and you might feel distracted and agitated. This period of time may be unpleasant, but eventually your body will figure out that it's not getting high doses of sugar spikes throughout the day, and it will stabilize and adjust to your new eating habits. Have some patience and trust the process. You'll be better off in the long run.

Outsmarting Hunger and Staying on Track

Hunger is a tricky thing. In general, there are two main types of hunger: emotional hunger and physical hunger. Emotional hunger is very common, and very hard to recognize. You may find yourself feeling hungry if you are bored, upset, stressed, happy, craving something . . . there are many triggers for emotional hunger. Physical hunger is your body actually telling you it needs nutrients, not a simple craving. Physical hunger can't be controlled; after all, if you go a long period of time without eating, your body will be quick to let you know. Emotional hunger, while more common for many, is also the worst kind, as you will be tempted to eat all sorts of food you really don't need. It's important to learn how to recognize emotional hunger, and learn what you can do to help control it.

There are a few basic tricks you can use to help you learn to feel the difference between emotional hunger and physical hunger. The first is to simply go a long time without eating one day—try to hold off until mid-afternoon, dinner, or as long as you can. Those afternoon hours will definitely be tough, and you'll notice physical signs of hunger that won't go away. It's best to do this when you can stay busy, so you aren't thinking about food—and don't worry, it's perfectly safe to do as long as you drink plenty of water. Not only is this a good exercise in self-control, but you'll learn what true physical hunger feels like.

ALERT

The cause of hunger can extend beyond emotional cravings and physical hunger. If you are very tired, stressed, upset about something, and especially if you are dehydrated, your body can become very hungry, and in these situations, it's even harder to resist. Try to get adequate sleep, take steps to reduce any chronic stressors, and drink plenty of water. You want to make this dieting process as easy as possible.

You'll never be able to fully eliminate hunger while trying to lose weight, and while in a caloric restriction. You'll need to be eating less food to lose fat, so chances are you'll just have to deal with being hungry at times. However, with the previous tricks, you can make it a whole lot easier on yourself, and hopefully you can learn the difference between needing food and wanting food. It's not going to be easy, but it's absolutely worth the effort to learn how to interpret the signs your body gives you.

Improving Your Hormonal Profile

Managing your carbohydrate intake can have positive impacts on your hormonal profile as well, especially if it leads to a reduction in body fat. As discussed earlier, insulin management is very important for a whole host of things. Controlling carbohydrate intake can also be beneficial to sex hormone production, mainly testosterone and estrogen. If you are a following a diet plan that recommends a reduced carbohydrate intake, you will most likely be eating more healthy fats as part of the plan, to make up for the caloric deficit created from removing the carbs. Hormonal functioning is very complex, but increasing your healthy dietary fat intake and stabilizing blood sugar can help support healthy hormone levels in both men and women.

Building a Caloric Deficit for Fat Loss

To lower body fat levels, you must be in a caloric deficit. There is no way around this. Everyone's metabolism is different, so everyone has different caloric needs, but if you are not expending more calories than you are eating, you will not be able to lose fat. With that being said, there are several strategies that can be used to get yourself into the needed caloric deficit for weight loss.

Build a Caloric Deficit with Food

The simplest way to create a caloric deficit is to eat less food. If you are taking in 2,500 calories per day, reducing your intake to 2,000 is a great place to start, and should be pretty manageable. It's nothing drastic, and by replacing some high-calorie foods with some lower-calorie, more filling foods such as fibrous vegetables and lean proteins, you should be able to control your hunger as well. If you don't have time to exercise, don't know how, or just want a simple way to start your fat-loss journey, the first step should always be to simply eat less food.

A quick and easy way to create a caloric deficit, if you are new to dieting, is to stop drinking liquid calories. Soft drinks, fruit juice, fancy coffee drinks—all of these can be loaded with calories that don't fill you up at all. Try to drink only zero-calorie beverages for a while, and depending on your previous drinking habits, you may find that this alone is enough to start the fat-loss process.

The exact number may vary from person to person, but generally speaking, a pound of fat is roughly 3,500 calories. If you can stay in a deficit of 500 calories per day, that would equate to roughly 1 pound of fat lost per week, which is a very sustainable and healthy rate of weight loss. The numbers may not always work out perfectly, and a lot of other factors can influence your weight on the scale. Regardless, it's easy to see how eating fewer calories each day is an easy way to lose fat.

Build a Caloric Deficit with Exercise

The second way to create a caloric deficit is by increasing your physical activity. All functions of life use calories for energy, from getting up and making breakfast to going for a run, and everything in between. By increasing your energy output each day, you can help create a deficit and burn more calories.

NEAT, or non-exercise activity thermogenesis, refers to the calories burned from any activity that isn't specifically exercise. So if you don't want to run or go to the gym, there are plenty of ways you can still increase your daily energy output. Park farther away from your destination when you go places and walk more, try to stand up periodically throughout the day and move around if you find yourself sitting a lot—the options are endless. You want to do something to get up and get moving, but it doesn't have to be something you don't enjoy.

The one issue with using exercise to create a deficit is trying to figure out how many calories you are actually burning. Every single person is different, so using calories-burned calculators and other tools may not be the most accurate method. It's a start, but it won't be perfect. It's also important to note that as you get better at things, or more efficient, it takes less energy to perform the action. You might go for a long walk around the neighborhood and feel pretty exhausted, but if you do this same walk every day, after a few weeks you'll be burning many fewer calories than when you started. Rather than try to calculate how many calories you burned when you do something, just try to move more every day and enjoy the process, realizing you are taking care of your body and making it function better.

Build a Deficit with Both Nutrition and Exercise

The single most efficient way to create the caloric deficit needed to lose fat is to use a combination of both diet and exercise to reach your goals. You could get by with just one or the other, but since both a healthy diet and regular exercise have so many health benefits, there is no reason to leave one on the table. The two will work together to make you stronger and healthier, and help you reach your weight-loss goals in a safe way. By having a regular, challenging exercise plan in place, making an effort to move more whenever you can, and following a healthy meal plan that provides you the appropriate amount of calories for your goals, you can be sure you are doing everything in your power to set yourself up for success.

If you are exercising on a regular basis, be careful not to eat extra food to make up for it, thinking you earned it. A vigorous 30-minute workout may burn 250–300 calories, which is a great accomplishment, but it's all too easy to eat those calories right back up, even with something that may seem healthy. If you are exercising regularly you will be able to eat more overall than if you were sedentary, but be smart about it. On the flip side, if you overeat, don't try to burn it all off through exercise and punish yourself; you'll be miserable. Just lower your calories for the next few days and get right back on track.

In the end, all that matters is creating a consistent caloric deficit. Some weeks you'll find yourself more physically active and may be able to enjoy a little more food, and some weeks you'll probably have a little less activity and eat a little less—there is no right or wrong way to go about it. Try your best, get back on track if you slip up, and always remember that you're in this for the long haul and consistency is all that really matters.

Enjoying the Foods You Like—in Moderation!

The last main benefit of cycling your carbohydrates is also the most fun—you can still enjoy the foods you like in moderation, and not feel restricted. While you won't be eating bottomless pizza and pasta on a regular basis, when special occasions come up, or when you feel like indulging, you can make these foods fit into your plan. Speaking strictly in terms of fat loss, all that matters is the caloric deficit. On a high-carb day, if you spend some of those carbs on a treat you enjoy, you can still see results.

Think of your daily calorie and macronutrient limits as a bank account, and the amount of calories you should eat in a given day is how much money you have available to spend. If it's a low-carb day and you only have 100 grams of total carbohydrates for the day, chances are you probably don't want to use 80 of them on a bag of candy or piece of cake. You could do this, but then you'll have a much harder time going carb-less the rest of the day. However, if it's a high-carb day and you want to save some of them for dessert, that's completely acceptable.

If it seems wrong that you can enjoy sweets in moderation and still lose weight, just remind yourself of the science. There are healthier choices, sure, but as long as your total calories stay the same and allow you to stay under your caloric limit, there's no harm in enjoying something fun here and there.

You need to have self-control and be sure that one cookie doesn't turn into the whole box, but if you can learn to do that, you'll find this diet much more sustainable for the long run. It's much better to treat yourself from time to time than to try to completely eliminate all of the foods you enjoy until you reach your breaking point. If having an occasional treat helps you stay on your nutrition plan, then by all means, enjoy it. Life is meant to be enjoyed, after all, and this method of dieting can help you find that balance and enjoyment as you progress through your fat-loss journey.

CHAPTER 3

How to Get Started

Now that you know the science behind carbohydrate cycling, the benefits, and the reasons why it works so well, it's time to dig into the practical side and start planning your new diet. You need to figure out how to schedule your high- and low-carb days, how many carbohydrates you should be eating on those days, and how to plan for success. All of that will be covered in this chapter, which is your guide to assembling your first carbohydrate cycling plan.

Scheduling High-Carb and Low-Carb Days

The first step is to decide when you are going to have high-carbohydrate days and when you are going to have low-carbohydrate days. There are a couple of ways to go about figuring this out, and several factors that will influence your decisions. Personal preference also has a role in figuring this out. Carbohydrate cycling is a theory or practice, not a rigid, strict diet plan. You can set up your plan to fit your life, your schedule, and your preferences, and it will still be effective.

The first factor to consider is how many high-carb days you will have each week. Generally, this sort of plan works best when you have between two and four high-carb days, two if you aren't very active and four if you are very active, though personal preference and dieting history are also factors. If this is the first time you've ever tried to follow a diet plan, start with four high days and gradually lower them. If you've been dieting for a while and are stuck with some stubborn fat, you'll probably want to start with two or three high-carb days.

Scheduling Your Days If You Aren't a Regular Exerciser

If you aren't doing a lot of physical exercise on a regular basis, then the days you choose for your high-carb days are a matter of personal preference. It's best to not have them back-to-back, so you should try to spread them around the week. Consider your weekly schedule and social life. If you like to go out on the weekends for dinner and drinks, you may want to have Friday or Saturday be a high-carb day, with the other ones spread around the weekdays. Perhaps there's a night of the week where you join your work friends for a social outing, in which case you may want that to be a high-carb day. Ultimately, it will come down to convenience and what works best for you.

Scheduling Your Days If You Are a Regular Exerciser

If you do engage in physical exercise on a weekly basis, then you'll want to consider a few factors when planning your days. Physical exercise includes any exercise you do for 30 minutes or more with a moderate to high intensity level. If you go to the gym to lift weights, go for a long run, or participate in a long hike or fitness class, those would be exercise days. Intense exercise depletes glycogen and primes your body to absorb nutrients. Low-intensity activities such as slow, leisurely walking—for example walking around the mall—don't have the same effect.

ESSENTIAL

When you utilize resistance training at the proper intensity and really push yourself, you create an environment where your body will be more inclined to use nutrients for recovery and repair, rather than storing them as fat. Resistance training causes micro-damage to your muscles, so those few hours after a training session are a great time to enjoy your carbohydrates, as your body will use them to recover.

If you follow an exercise plan, then you'll want to have your high-carb days on your most physically active days, as those days have the greatest need for fuel in the form of glucose. You'll use glucose to exercise, and you'll use it to help your body recover, so it's a great time for higher carbohydrate intake. The timing of your food doesn't matter as much as some might claim, so don't go rushing home to eat immediately after exercising, but over the course of the day you should have a higher intake.

If your plan is three days per week of weight training, which is a good beginner-to-intermediate plan, make those your high-carb days. If you only train once or twice per week, you can choose where the third high-carb day will go. Not all exercise plans are three days, so if you are a following a four-, five-, or even six-day-per-week program, or if you have a highly active job, you'll have to do some thinking. Think about which of those days are the most physically exhausting for you, or the hardest to recover from, and use those days as your high-carb days. If you resistance train, for example, generally a lower-body workout is much more taxing than an arm or shoulder workout would be. Use those carbs to fuel your most intense activity.

Determining Your Intake Levels

Now it's time to figure out exactly how much food you need to eat on a daily basis. It's very important to realize that no calculation or estimation will ever be 100 percent accurate. Every person is unique, and this includes metabolic rates as well. These calculations may be very accurate for some people but way too high or low for others. However, for most people they are a good starting point. It can all get a little tricky, so grab a pencil and paper and get ready to do some calculations. There are calculators online that work well, but here you'll learn how to do it manually.

FACT

To get the most accurate idea of how many calories you need to eat each day, try logging your food intake for a week and see what happens. Pick a total caloric number, such as the one you'll calculate in the following section, and try to hit that number as close as you can each day for a week. This may require some precise tracking. If you lose weight, you're eating under your maintenance. If your weight doesn't change, you've found your maintenance level. If you gain weight, you are eating too much.

Step 1: Calculate Your Total Calories

To start, you'll want to find a total caloric intake goal for yourself. Again, this will just be a guess, but it may get you close. A good guideline is to take your total body weight and multiply it by 12 if you are sedentary and 14 if you are physically active on a regular basis. To be physically active you should either perform a manual labor job or spend at least three to four days per week doing moderate- to high-intensity activity. As an example, a 180-pound male, multiplying by 14 because he recently began an exercise program, would arrive at 2,520 calories ($180 \times 14 = 2,520$). Again, this may need to be adjusted up or down depending on how he responds, but it's a good starting point.

Step 2: Calculate Your Daily Protein Needs

Now that you have your total caloric intake, it's time to break it down into macronutrients. Remember, both a single gram of protein and a gram of carbohydrate have 4 calories, while a gram of fat has 9 calories. It's a good idea to aim for anywhere between 0.6–1 gram of protein per pound of body weight, aiming for the higher end if you are a regular exerciser. This may be the most important macronutrient, and the one that doesn't change on a daily basis. For the original example, 1 gram per pound would equal 180 grams each day, or 720 calories ($180 \times 4 = 720$).

As previously mentioned, protein along with carbs is needed to recover, it builds muscle, keeps you full, and is also very hard to digest. There is a factor called the TEF factor, or thermic effect of food. This refers to the amount of energy it takes to break down and absorb the food you eat. That's right—even the act of digesting your food burns calories. Protein has the highest TEF factor, so you'll burn the most calories from digestion by eating protein. This, combined with the fact that it keeps you full, makes it invaluable when on a diet.

Step 3: Calculate Your Carbohydrate and Fat Needs

At this point, how you distribute your remaining calories between carbohydrates and fat is largely a matter of personal preference. It's a good idea to have at least 20 percent of your total caloric intake come from fat, as it's essential for many functions in the body. There is no minimum for carbohydrate intake.

ALERT

When calculating your macronutrient needs, always remember the total calorie conversions. 1 gram protein = 4 calories. 1 gram carbohydrate = 4 calories. 1 gram fat = 9 calories. It's very easy to forget this and count fat calories as 4 as well, so be careful and double-check your numbers.

Let's get back to our example 180-pound male. If you recall, his total caloric needs were 2,520, with 720 of them being dedicated to protein each day. This leaves him with exactly 1,800 remaining calories to distribute as he sees best. If fat is to be kept at a minimum of 20 percent, some math can help him with the rest. Twenty percent of 2,520, the total calorie goal, is 504 total calories. To convert that to grams of fat, he'll divide this number by 9, as fat has 9 calories per gram. This gives him 56 grams of fat at minimum each day. If you got lost there, take your total calories each day, multiply it by 0.2, and then take whatever number you get, and divide it by 9.

ESSENTIAL

He now has 180 grams of protein, 56 grams of fat, and the remaining calories are from carbohydrates. On a high-carb day, fat would stay low, around 56–60 grams, and the rest would be carbs. On a low-carb day, fat may increase to a fairly high amount. If total calories are 2,520, with the 180 protein and 56 fat established, that leaves 324 grams of carbohydrates for a high-carb day. On a low-carb day, if the carbohydrates were lowered to 200 grams, that would add an extra 55 grams of fat, bringing his daily total as high as 110. Remember, total calories should stay the same, and protein should stay the same, so if you lower carbs, you'll have to increase fat to reach your total caloric needs.

If you got lost, here is a quick recap of all the steps:

- Multiply your body weight by 12–14 to get total caloric needs (12 for less active people, 14 for more active people).
- Eat 0.6–1 gram of protein per pound of body weight; multiply this by 4 to get total protein calories.
- Multiply the total number from step 1 by 0.2 to get your minimum fat calories.
- Subtract your protein calories from your total calories, and the remaining calories can be split between carbohydrates and fat as you see fit.

Step 4: Set Your Carb Numbers for High and Low Days

This comes down to personal preference, and how your body responds. Some people can have very high carb intakes and get very lean, and some need to keep their intake very low to lose fat. It will take some experimenting and trial and error to see how you respond best. Take note of how you feel in terms of energy, mood, and recovery on low and high days, and adjust as needed.

To start with a rough guess, aim for 1–1.5 grams of carbohydrate per pound of body weight on your high days and 0.5 gram per pound or less on your low days. On low days, depending on how low your carbs actually end up, you may be limited to just the trace carbs you'll find in vegetables, and that's okay.

Meal Planning: Your Key to Success

The key to successfully hitting your goals each day is to plan ahead. As long as you stay within your caloric intake goals, you'll see results. If you can go even further and stay pretty close to your total protein, carb, and fat goals, you'll see even better results. However, if you don't plan ahead, you'll have a very hard time hitting your goals with any sort of accuracy, and most likely you'll end up running out of a nutrient or getting close to your caloric limit before you are done eating for the day.

ESSENTIAL

If you have a family to care for or an unpredictable schedule, it can be hard to follow any sort of plan with consistency. The best thing to do is to try to automate as many meals as you can, and keep them a constant. If you really don't think you can handle planning, you may want to use some sort of calorie tracking app, so that you always have an idea of where you are at as you go through each day.

The best thing to do is spend some time creating a meal plan that allows you to stay within your calories, and try to eat as close to that plan as you can. It can be a lot of work up front, but once you have a written plan in front of you, following it is much easier than tracking as you go each day and adjusting on the fly. You'll want to come up with a few sample days of eating, for high- and low-carb days. This way, even if something comes up and you are unable to follow the plan exactly, you'll have a rough idea of what your whole day should look like, and you can plan ahead. If you know you'll have a lot of carbs for dinner, you can just look at your plan and take those carbs out of other meals to save them.

Food Shopping and Preparation

Grocery shopping ahead of time and preparing meals in advance are essential to your success, especially if you have a busy schedule. There's nothing worse than being very hungry, not having the food you need around, and then having to choose between going to the store or ordering takeout. You'll need a lot of willpower in that situation, so it's best to just plan ahead.

As you go about creating your meal plan, think about meals that are convenient to prepare and enjoyable for you. The recipes and sample meal plans in the back of this book will be very helpful in your planning. Once you have your plan in place, it's easy to make a grocery list of what you'll need to prepare your food, and spend a few hours cooking it all and storing it for reheating later. If you have a flexible schedule with no commitments, you may be able to prepare your meals fresh as you go, but there's nothing wrong with cooking all your food at once and reheating as you need it.

ALERT

If you end up eating out a lot because of a busy schedule, work, running errands, or anything else, you may want to consider finding a few healthy options ahead of time at the places you know you'll go. If you work across from a café that you find yourself frequenting for lunch throughout the week, do some investigation and see if you can find their nutrition information, and a meal that you can fit into your daily plan. There's nothing wrong with eating out and enjoying food if you can make it fit.

By planning ahead, shopping, and spending some time cooking, you can be sure that you have all the meals ready to go. You have a plan, and you have the food; all you need now is the willpower and self-discipline to execute the plan and follow through.

Good and Bad Nutrient Combos

For the most part, you can technically eat any foods you want, whenever you want, and still see results if the calories and macronutrients are right. However, there is a big difference between something working and something being optimal. When planning your meals, there are a few nutrient combinations to consider, and one in particular you want to avoid. First, remember that carbohydrates trigger your body to release insulin, and insulin flips the switch that turns your body into storage mode. If carbohydrates are in the meal, that meal will be absorbed and stored very quickly.

As you might be able to guess, it is important that you are careful with how you plan your meals if you want to optimize your progress. By eating carbohydrates and proteins together, such as after a workout, you are able to absorb and store the protein and carbs quickly, which is something you want. Protein and fats together is a good option when you want to stay full for a while. They both digest slowly, and the slow digestion will help give your body time to use them appropriately, rather than rushing to store them in the most readily available place, which is your fat.

The one combination you'll want to consider avoiding is carbohydrates and fat. If you have to combine them, it won't be the worst thing in the world—it isn't going to cause you to gain instant weight or derail your progress. However, for optimal performance, it's probably best to avoid this combination when possible, or at least keep fat low. If you raise your insulin, which makes your body want to store nutrients, and all you have floating around is glucose and fatty acids, chances are those will go straight to your fat cells. Again, you can still see results in the long term, but this probably isn't a combination you want on a regular basis.

Scheduling "Cheat" Meals

Straying off your plan because you didn't have self-control and ate way too much food isn't optimal. You can get back on track, so there's no need to beat yourself up over it, but it's not going to help you reach your goals any faster. The beauty of this plan is that just about any food you want can be made to fit; you just have to use moderation.

If you want dessert, or sweets, or a slice of pizza, it's more than okay to indulge every so often; in fact, it's probably good for your sanity so you don't go crazy from resisting your favorite foods all the time. Just make sure you plan ahead. Tell yourself you'll enjoy it without feeling guilty, enjoy your treat, and get back on the program. If you don't have the self-control to stop with just a small portion, you may not want to go off plan too much, but if you can handle it without eating everything in sight, then go for it.

ESSENTIAL

Always remember that it's okay to enjoy life, and you shouldn't feel guilty, especially if you plan ahead. If you start to feel guilty, it's easy to bring yourself down, and the temptation to just give up entirely is much stronger. Plan ahead, and there's no need for guilt. Even if you do slip up accidentally, just brush it off and get back on track the next day.

Tips and Tricks to Maximize Your Results

There are a few tricks and tips you can implement that can help you reach your goals faster and make the whole process seem easier. These tips aren't anything magical, but as you get used to following your plan, develop some consistent habits, and feel comfortable with what you are doing, these little tricks can help take things to the next level.

Eat Most of Your Carbohydrates Before and After Your Workouts

If you are active, it's a good idea to eat a large portion of your carbohydrates around your workout, anywhere from 30–50 percent, if not more. When you are pushing your body hard, you need proper fuel to perform at the highest level, and carbs will help you do this. After a tough workout, your body will tend to use any food you consume for recovery and repair, so if you are really working hard, any food you eat within an hour or two of your workout will most likely go to a useful cause, rather than being stored as fat. If you want to have a high-carb meal, or plan a cheat meal, right after a tough strength-training session is the perfect time.

Add Green Vegetables to Every Meal

Green fibrous vegetables are a really great way to add volume and fiber to your food, without adding a whole lot of calories. Broccoli, spinach, kale, lettuce, and anything else green would be good choices. If you find yourself really dropping your calories low to work off those last few stubborn pounds, chances are you'll feel hungry throughout the day. Eating large portions of greens with your meals will go a long way toward keeping you full.

Drink Plenty of Water with and Between Meals

Water is the most essential thing you consume. It's also very common to feel like you are hungry when your body is actually thirsty and needs hydration. The two signals are very similar, and hard to distinguish between. A good rule is to drink a large glass of water with each meal, and sip water throughout the day between meals. If you don't enjoy drinking plain water, try using fresh lemon, lime, or other fruit to add some flavor, or try carbonated, flavored, zero-calorie waters.

CHAPTER 4

Advanced Carb Cycling Strategies

At some point, you may run into sticking points, or plateaus, while on your carb cycling journey. As you get leaner, you may have to employ some fancy tricks to keep the results coming. Once you have mastered the basics of carb cycling, there are several advanced steps you can take to keep things moving and raise your results to the next level. These strategies probably wouldn't be appropriate for someone who has just started a diet, but will work well if you've reached a certain level of leanness and find yourself stuck.

Adding Exercise

Carb cycling can be very effective in and of itself. Regardless of your current health and fitness levels, cycling your carb intake can improve your body composition, mood, and a whole host of other health benefits. However, as you progress along your journey, you will probably run into sticking points, or plateaus. When these situations happen, there are a few advanced strategies and tips you can implement to get things moving again.

Without a doubt, adding exercise to your daily life is the most efficient way to lose body fat, increase a vast number of health markers, such as lowered blood pressure and improved cholesterol levels, and avoid plateauing as you seek improved body composition. There are so many ways to get active; it doesn't have to be limited to going to the gym and working out or going for a run. Find something you enjoy, and work to make it a habit over time.

ESSENTIAL

All activities of human life burn calories. Eating, sleeping, digesting food, walking—it doesn't have to be exercise for the sake of exercise, if that isn't your cup of tea. It's best to make a point of just moving around more throughout the day, as often as you can. Whether it's going for a walk around the neighborhood, taking the stairs instead of the escalator, or trying a new sport, every little bit adds up. Using a pedometer or activity tracker can be a fun, motivating way to set daily goals for yourself and try to hit them.

When beginning an exercise program, you should start slowly if you aren't used to regular physical activity. Start with two to three times per week, for half an hour or so, and go from there. You want to pace yourself; exercise should fit into your life, not make you stressed and burned out. Remember, you're in this for the long haul, so there is no need to rush anything. Before starting any exercise program, always check with your doctor to make sure you're cleared for that level of physical activity.

Endurance Training versus Strength Training

So you've decided to pick up an exercise routine; now it's time to figure out exactly what it is you plan on doing. Typically, when it comes to working out, you'll likely see endurance training and strength training as the two main types marketed for fat loss. While strength and endurance training have some overlap, overall they are very different, and both have their place in a well-rounded fitness program.

FACT

Endurance training may bring to mind long-distance marathon runners or triathletes, but it can be anything that trains your cardiovascular system. By improving your cardiovascular system, you will improve the health of your heart and lungs and make your body more efficient at transporting oxygen and nutrients. Endurance training can be biking, rowing, swimming, walking, playing sports, running sprints, or any other activity that elevates your heart rate for an extended period of time.

Endurance training, or cardio, is generally included in a program to improve cardiovascular system health and burn calories. While you are active, your heart rate is elevated, you'll be burning more calories than usual, and your cardiovascular system will be working hard, making it stronger and more efficient in the long run. After the activity, your body will gradually cool down, returning to its normal state. During the activity itself, endurance training generally burns more calories than strength training, which is why so many begin running or walking to lose weight.

ALERT

It's very important to look at exercise as improving your body's health—because it is. If you see it as punishment or strictly as a way to burn calories, you will be less likely to enjoy it and to make it a sustainable habit. Remember, you are getting stronger, and setting yourself up to live a longer, healthier life. Burning extra calories is just a nice side effect.

With strength training, there are many variables that come into play, but the effects are usually a little bit different from endurance training. Your heart rate will be elevated, sure, but the amount of rest you take between your workout sets and the total amount of work you do will have an impact. Strength training improves body composition by increasing lean muscle mass over time, and with the proper intensity it has a strong positive impact on your hormones as well. It can also improve posture, reduce pain, and strengthen your bones when done over a long period of time.

Beginning an Endurance Training Program

Before beginning any exercise program, always consult with your doctor. Exercise is stressful on your body, and if you have any conditions involving your heart or respiratory system, you may have specific limits in place. Once you have your doctor's clearance, it's time to get started.

Remember, the most important thing is to start very slowly and build your way up over time. Pushing yourself too hard, especially when just beginning a new routine, can be very unpleasant. You need to work hard, but at a level that is appropriate for you. If you're just starting, try to do 20–30 minutes twice a week of any activity. It can be walking, riding your bike, going for a hike, using a rowing machine at the gym—whatever you prefer. Rather than get into fancy heart-rate calculations or anything like that, just aim to go at a pace that challenges you, but not to the point of being unable to finish. If you can hold a full conversation, it's probably too easy. However, if you are breathing so hard you can't form a sentence without getting dizzy, that's too much. Aim for somewhere in the middle.

If you're more advanced and are used to going on long jogs or running on a regular basis, you'll need to find ways to increase your intensity. Your body becomes efficient at things over time, so if you started out exercising with 2-mile jogs, which may seem incredibly difficult at first, eventually they will feel easy, and you won't burn as many calories or see the same benefits. If you're an advanced endurance trainee, you'll need to either add more time to your workouts or increase the intensity. Running hills, using interval training, or increasing the resistance on a bike or elliptical are all good ways to increase your intensity. Always be sure you are challenging yourself appropriately.

As you improve your fitness levels over time, you should look to increase your weekly endurance training volume if you get stuck and feel you need more activity. If fat loss slows, you can either eat less food or burn more calories. If you want to burn more calories, you can just figure out how much cardio you are doing each week and do a little more. You can add 5–10 minutes to each session or add an extra cardio workout, but your goal should be to do a little more over the course of the week. It's more practical and easier to do a little more each day rather than try to do all of your cardio in one long session.

QUESTION

Is HIIT training, or interval training, beneficial?
HIIT training stands for high-intensity interval training. If you can't guess from the name, this type of training is very challenging, and should only be used by intermediate to advanced trainees. If you've been doing endurance training for a while and want to step up your game, intervals are a great way to do this. You could choose short intervals with higher intensities, such as fast sprints for 10–20 seconds, or longer intervals at lower intensities, something like a 1-minute jog with a 1-minute walk for recovery. Another example would be running at your top speed for 10 seconds, and then resting or walking slowly for 1 minute before repeating. To see sample interval workouts you can try, visit *www.theathleticphysique.com/carb-cycling-book*.

Strength-Training Workouts

The number of strength-training workouts available can be overwhelming. When starting out, all you need is a well-rounded full-body workout, which you can do two to three times per week. Down the road you can look into different training splits and routines, but for now, just figure out a good routine that works all the major muscle groups, and perform it to the best of your ability.

Strength training doesn't always have to involve weights or weight machines. You can get a very challenging training effect using just your body weight and basic equipment you have available at home, such as chairs and steps. If you prefer to be outdoors, you can work out at a park, beach, or even a playground. Joining a traditional gym is not necessary. It can be beneficial depending on your goals, but you can also get great results without ever setting foot in a gym.

The following workouts can be performed two to three times per week, and you should give yourself at least one day off in between, to rest and recover.

Sample Home Workouts

Joining a gym is great, but it can be expensive or inconvenient. If it's an option for you, it's a great tool to take advantage of, but if you are unable to join a gym for any reason, you can still use exercise and strength training to really push yourself to the next level. Here are some basic bodyweight workouts you can do anywhere—if you have space to move, you can do these workouts.

ESSENTIAL

These workouts are designed for all fitness levels; for each exercise, there is a variation to make it harder, and a variation to make it easier. For this book, all exercises are text only. If you'd like to see more detailed instructions for the workouts, as well as photo demonstrations of all the exercises, please visit *www.theathleticphysique.com/ carb-cycling-book*, a site created to go along with this book.

There are two options for the following workouts: a three-days-per-week beginner plan and a four-days-per-week intermediate plan. It's best to start with three days and go up from there. With the beginner plan, you'll have three full-body workouts to complete over the course of the week; any days will work as long as you don't do two back-to-back days. With the four-day plan, you'll have two upper body days and two lower-body days. You can do an upper and lower back-to-back, but then you should take at least a day off to rest and recover.

Full-Body Beginner's Workout

With this workout, you should complete all exercises in order, as quickly as you can. Warm up by doing jumping jacks, a brisk walk or jog, or anything else to get your heart going for around 5 minutes before the workout. There is also a more detailed warmup on the website, along with easier and harder versions of each exercise. Try to rest for no more than 15–20 seconds in between. At the end of the workout, rest up to 2 minutes, until you feel recovered, then repeat the whole circuit. Start by doing two rounds of the workout, and after one week, bump it up to three total rounds.

- Bodyweight Squats × 15
- Push-ups × 10
- Reverse Lunges × 10 per leg
- Plank × 30 seconds
- Superman × 15
- Glute Bridge × 15
- Bird Dog × 8 per side

Once you've reached the point where this feels too easy, you can move up to the intermediate workouts. All of these workouts should be fairly quick once you learn the exercises, so if you feel like adding more, it wouldn't hurt to go for a walk, jog, hike, or some other cardio activity after you are finished.

Intermediate Workout

Just like the beginner's workout, you should complete all exercises in order, as quickly as you can. Move between exercises quickly; at the end, rest until you feel recovered, then repeat the whole circuit. You should be aiming for three total rounds to start. If you want to make it more challenging, simply decrease the amount of rest you take between rounds. Remember to visit the website for easier and harder versions of each exercise.

UPPER-BODY WORKOUT

- Push-Ups × 25
- Superman × 20
- Side Plank × 30 seconds per side
- Burpees × 10
- Reverse Crunch × 20
- Chair or Bench Dips × 15

LOWER-BODY WORKOUT

- Bodyweight Squats × 25
- Side Lunges × 15 per leg
- Glute Bridge × 25
- Split Squats × 15 per leg
- Side Lying Hip Raises × 20 per leg
- Reverse Lunges × 20 per leg

Once you've reached the point where the intermediate workouts feel too easy, it may be time to consider investing in some exercise equipment or a gym membership. There are certain muscle groups that can be challenging to train without any equipment, so if you find that you enjoy working out and want to do more, a gym may be your best option. You can also find boot camps, workout classes, or many other fitness-related group activities to enjoy that can mix things up and challenge you.

Cycling Carbs Around Your Workouts

Planning your week so that your high-carb days fall on your training days is a very effective way to get the best possible results. Purposefully exercising and pushing your body requires a lot more energy than simply walking around and going about your daily tasks. The body's preferred fuel source for exercise is glycogen, as it is the easiest to convert to useable energy. Glycogen comes from carbohydrates, which means that on workout days there's a good chance that the carbs you eat will be used to fuel your workout and/or help you recover from it. On days when you aren't training hard, you don't need as many carbs to function, which is why it is best to have high-carb days on your workout days.

If you really want to take this a step further, it's worth taking a look at your nutrient timing, or your eating schedule. Ultimately, weight loss is controlled by total calories, so even if you don't follow a set eating plan, you can still see great results if you consume the proper amount of food each day. Timing your food intake, however, especially your carbohydrate intake, can absolutely improve both the quality of your workouts and your recovery from them, and can help ensure that the food you eat is used for maximum efficiency. It's an advanced strategy that enables you to give your body the greatest chance at using carbohydrates effectively, rather than storing them as body fat.

ALERT

It's not bad to have carbs on non-workout days, and they don't make you fat, regardless of what you may hear. If you want to carb cycle and don't follow an exercise routine, you'll still want to have higher-carb days. As long as your total calories remain the same, you'll be just fine, so don't be scared to eat carbohydrates even if you aren't exercising.

A good way to experiment with this is to put about half of your total daily carb intake around your workout. If you've figured out that you will be consuming 200 grams on a workout day, take at least 100 of those grams and eat half before and the other half after your workout. Not only are carbohydrates used for fuel, but they are also very important for recovery. As you eat carbs, insulin spikes, which helps your body push nutrients into the muscles faster, resulting in improved recovery. Stick with simple carbs that will be easy to digest, such as fruit, rice, potatoes, and pasta. The exact timing isn't super important, but you should try to eat your pre- and post-workout carbs within one to two hours of beginning or ending your workout.

Breaking Through Fat-Loss Plateaus

If you've reached the point where you exercise regularly, and you have your high-carb days on your training days, and you're eating your carbs around your workouts, you may still find yourself getting stuck in your weight-loss journey. If you are trying to reach very low levels of body fat and find yourself stalling, or struggling, here are a few more advanced strategies you may want to consider. They won't work for everyone, as people have different food preferences and carbohydrate tolerances, but they are worth trying.

Multilevel Carb Cycling

If you've steadily followed the basic template for a while, with high days and low days, it may be time to start adding an intake somewhere in the middle to vary it even more. For example, you may have your high days set at 200 grams and your low days set at 75 grams. If this has stopped working, you may be able to get things moving again by really driving down those low-carb numbers and adding a middle number. You might have 25-gram days, 100-gram days, and 200-gram days now, rather than simply high or low. The schedule could look something like this:

- Sunday: 25 grams carbs
- Monday: 25 grams carbs
- Tuesday: 25 grams carbs
- Wednesday: 100 grams carbs
- Thursday: 25 grams carbs
- Friday: 25 grams carbs
- Saturday: 200 grams carbs

As you can see, with a schedule like this, you'd have two blocks of low-carb days followed by high-carb, or re-feed, days. Varying your totals in such a way allows you to lower your overall caloric intake and get all the benefits of having low carbohydrate intake for those few days. Remember, this is an advanced strategy, so there is no need to start with such low-carb days unless you've been stuck for some time and can't find any other way to break your plateau.

When you use this method, you should keep your protein and fat roughly the same on all of the days. Remember, by keeping your carbohydrate intake so low (at 25 grams), most of the carbs you will be eating will be trace carbs from fruits and vegetables, therefore your calories will be very low. When you raise your carbs on your mid- and high-carb days, your caloric intake will increase, but this is perfectly fine. As long as you are in a caloric deficit for the whole week, you'll still see results.

The Weekly Depletion and Re-Feed

This advanced method puts all of your high carbohydrate intake on the weekend, or whatever two consecutive days you choose, and lets you stay in a low-carb state all week. Many people have found success by staying disciplined with their diet during the week, then allowing themselves the weekend to have a very controlled re-feed period. By having your high-carb days on the weekend, you can be more accommodating of social events that involve food and treat yourself a little bit.

There may be physiological benefits to this method as well, not just the mental break. As you begin to get very lean, or if you've been dieting for a long period of time, your metabolism can adjust, and weight loss can begin to stall. If you've been working out hard and eating very restricted calories, then a sudden increase for a day or two can jolt your body into fat-burning mode again. If you've just begun a diet, you probably don't need re-feed (or higher calorie) days, but if you've been grinding away at it for a while, it may be just the thing you need. If you choose this method, you will benefit most by lowering your total calories on your lower-carb days, and raising your calories on your higher-carb, re-feed days. For example, if your daily average has been 2,000 calories, you could shift five low-carb days to 1,700 by lowering your carbs and fat, and your two re-feed days could be 2,750, with very high carb intake. This will still make your daily total for the week average out to 2,000.

ALERT

If you choose to use this method, or any other re-feed strategy, remember that carbohydrates make you hold water. If you deplete your glycogen stores over the week, you'll lose water weight. By increasing your carb intake for a day or two to refill your glycogen levels, you'll regain some of the water. No need to be alarmed if you see the scale jump after the re-feed days. If you stayed within your caloric limits, you'll be fine; it's most likely water weight.

Carb Back-Loading

The last advanced strategy is carb back-loading. This tends to help greatly with dietary adherence, and may be worth a try if you find yourself craving food and snacks late at night. The method is simple—save all of your carbs for the end of the day. It may seem counter-intuitive, and you've probably read that eating after a certain time of day makes you fat. There is absolutely no truth to this at all; all that matters is your total daily caloric intake.

With carb back-loading, you make sure your first meals and snacks are composed of primarily lean proteins and some fats and vegetables. For your last meal of the day, you'll have all the remaining carbs. This could be a big bowl of rice or pasta, crackers, chips, or anything else you like and enjoy. You are able to go to bed satisfied, you can reduce cravings, and if you love carbs, you give yourself something to look forward to at the end of each day.

CHAPTER 5

The Maintenance Phase

If you can find the willpower to stick with a solid nutrition and exercise program, you should have no problems reaching your fat-loss goal. It will take time, but if you can learn to enjoy the journey, it won't be so bad. However, one thing often overlooked when discussing diets is what to do once you hit your goal. If you go right back to your old habits, chances are you'll get your old body back. Many diets show dramatic before-and-after transformations, yet they don't tell you what happens to those people once they try to go back to a normal eating plan. You need to know how to transition from your caloric deficit phase to a normal, sustainable maintenance diet that allows you to keep and enjoy your new body. This chapter will show you how.

Do You Need to Carb Cycle Forever?

If you've reached your goal, you should have an opinion on carb cycling. You may love it or you may hate it, but hopefully it has helped you reach your goal without fully restricting or eliminating any food sources. At the end of a diet phase you'll need to find some way of eating that you will be able to follow, that is stress free, and that won't cause you to gain all your weight back within those first few weeks.

The beauty of carb cycling is that it doesn't necessarily mean you'll always need to be tracking food, measuring things, and eating in a caloric deficit. Once you have learned the principles of carb cycling and used them to reach your goal, they will have become your new dietary norm. It's a style of eating you can follow as long as you wish with no negative side effects. Cycling of your carbohydrate intake is probably one of the healthiest styles of eating you can follow. Even after you work back up to the point where you are eating a lot more food again, you can still reap all the health benefits of carb cycling, regardless of whether fat loss is a goal.

ESSENTIAL

Remember, carb cycling simply refers to varying your carbohydrate intake on a day-to-day basis. It does not necessarily mean fat loss or weight gain; it's just a method. You can be carb cycling without actively trying to lose weight; you can even carb cycle on a weight-gain plan.

With some practice, you may be able to reach the point where you can intuitively eat without obsessively measuring everything and still maintain a healthy weight. This could mean eating more carbs around your workouts with fewer on-off days and mindfully watching your portions the rest of the day without weighing everything you eat. Or you may find you enjoy the precision of tracking food and having the ability to adjust your intake at will to reach your weight goal. Either way, you can reach the point where you are eating the foods you enjoy on a regular basis and still maintain your new body; it just takes patience, self-control, and time.

Transitioning to a "Normal" Eating Style

Nobody wants to diet forever, so it's important to get back to a normal, or maintenance, level. Staying in a caloric deficit long-term can have several negative side effects. Your metabolism may slow down, thyroid activity can decrease, and the function and production of other hormones can be negatively affected. These effects are especially seen in those who have to bring their calories very low to lose fat and stay this way for a sustained period of time, such as when preparing for a photoshoot or physique contest. Returning to a maintenance level in an efficient way should be your first order of business after finishing a diet.

In addition to hormonal effects, you also have a greater chance of missing out on important nutrients if you are in a caloric deficit for a long time. Even if all of your dietary choices are unprocessed, nutritious, whole food sources, you're still going to be eating less of them.

The Importance of Reverse Dieting

Reverse dieting is a term that refers to increasing your caloric intake, slowly, over a given period of time. Remember, your body is very smart. Just as it adapts to running on decreased calories, which is why you may hit plateaus while dieting, your body can adjust to increased calories. By implementing slow, strategic raises in your food intake, you can increase your food intake over time without seeing a fast rebound and weight gain.

QUESTION

Why should I even bother with a reverse diet? I want to keep all the weight off!
You will keep most of your weight off, but chances are you won't be able to sustain the diet you used to reach your goal forever. It can be very time consuming and stressful trying to be very strict and controlled with your food intake. Reverse dieting helps you ease into a sustainable, easy way of eating for long-term health, so you can enjoy life and not have to worry about food all the time. Most people want to eat as much food as they can without gaining fat, and this allows you to do that!

The goal with reverse dieting is to very slowly increase your food intake, while minimizing fat gain, not completely eliminating it. As an example, if you begin a diet with a daily intake of 3,000 calories per day, lose 20 pounds, and end the diet eating 1,800 calories, you wouldn't be able to jump right back to 3,000 per day and keep all 20 pounds off. However, if you have the self-control to slowly and strategically increase your food over time, you may be able to get back to 3,000 calories and keep 15 of those pounds off, in which case you're in a much better place than when you started.

Here is an example of how this works. Let's say a 200-pound male who is eating around 3,500 calories per day wants to lose fat. Over the course of eight to ten months, he picks up a regular exercise routine, reduces his calories as he goes, and ends his diet eating 1,900 calories per day and weighing 175 pounds. This man now wants to stay around 175, but 1,900 calories is very low and will be hard to sustain for a long time, especially since he will continue exercising. If this man immediately starts consuming 3,500 calories again, chances are he'll gain most of that fat back very quickly. His body will be used to operating and running efficiently at 1,900, so with all this extra food added back in all at once, his body will probably store a lot of fat.

ESSENTIAL

Metabolic capacity refers to the number of calories your body runs on daily to maintain its current weight. If you eat 1,800 calories per day and your weight doesn't change week to week, that's your maintenance level. Through hard work and careful planning, you may be able to increase your body's metabolic capacity, allowing you to eat more food while maintaining your current weight. You can also decrease your capacity through long-term caloric restriction or a sedentary lifestyle.

Now, let's say this same man instead takes the slow approach. After finishing his diet, he increases his food from 1,900 to 1,950. He stays on this for a week or two, lets his body adapt, and then increases to 2,100. He might gain a pound or two from extra water, but if he keeps the food constant and continues to exercise, his body will probably rebalance itself back out around his new weight of 175.

If he continues adding very small increases every seven to fourteen days, he will be slowly building his metabolic capacity, or the amount of food he uses daily to function. Some weight gain may happen over time, but it's very possible this man could increase his food intake back to 3,500 over a few months and still be within 5 or so pounds of his new body weight.

This approach does take patience and discipline, but it's the best option post-diet, unless you want to be in the dieting mindset forever, or gain all of your weight back. So many diets fail to address what to do once you hit your goal; now you know. There is no need to throw away the results you've worked so hard for when you can learn to maintain them for the long run.

Carb Cycling for Maintenance and for Life

As was briefly mentioned before, once you've reached your goal weight and have been there for a while, giving your body time to adjust and learn how to maintain its current level of body fat, you can transition to a way of eating that doesn't require any special tracking. If you've reached your goal, you've probably learned how to stick to a plan without straying too far, and learned a little bit of self-control as well. You can use these new skills to eat mindfully and maintain your new, lean body forever.

ALERT

Take a look at what your eating habits were before you ever began this diet, and be honest with yourself. If you simply weren't aware of how you should be eating, then you can probably shift into a maintenance mode fairly easily. However, if you knew what sort of foods you should be eating and struggled more with self-control or binge eating, or couldn't avoid daily snacks and junk food, you may want to stick with tracking a little longer and slowly ease into instinctive eating.

The best way to go about this is to simply make your meals consist of lean proteins, vegetables, and low to moderate amounts of fat. On days you will be engaging in resistance training or high-intensity exercise, eat some carbs before and after. Rice, potatoes, fruit, or any other whole-food carb source is perfectly acceptable here. On top of this, maybe once or twice per week you should allow yourself to indulge a little. "Cheating" is not the most positive word, as this can imply an all-out eating session, but if you've been training hard and sticking to the plan, having one meal with moderate portions of foods you enjoy won't hurt you.

Here are some useful and quick visual measurements for you. It's not necessary to obsess over the exact measurements, but it is helpful to be able to quickly look at food and estimate how much a serving is. When building your meals, these are the guidelines that you should aim for.

- 1 serving lean protein per meal—About the size of the palm of your hand.
- 1–2 handfuls of vegetables per meal—Self-explanatory; roughly what you could scoop up with one or two hands.
- 1 small portion of fat with most meals—About the size of your thumb. For whole eggs, or fattier cuts of meat, no additional fat is needed.
- 1 fist-sized serving of carbohydrates pre- and post-workout—Most of your meals will now be very light on carbs. But the meals before and after your workout should each have a serving of carbs roughly the size of your fist. If you find you aren't recovering well from workouts, go with two servings post-workout.

When you look at the sample meal plans at the end of this book, you'll see workout days and rest days. Those days are set up in a way similar to what was just described: whole food choices, with carbohydrates around the workouts. You can eat whatever you like, as the plans are just samples, but they are good examples of how you could structure your daily meals. If you are choosing mostly whole-food sources and mindfully controlling your portion sizes, you shouldn't have much of an issue maintaining a healthy, lean body.

Instinctive Eating versus Carb Cycling

You can use general carb cycling to maintain your results. For some people this is easily sustainable, but others may not be able to follow this. Some households regularly consume rice or beans as a staple ingredient, or it may just not be convenient to eliminate carbs completely. You may just love carbs and want them daily. If this is the case, you can still maintain your results and eat carbs daily; you'll just have to be a bit more careful.

If you are carb cycling with whole foods and lean protein sources, just by their nature you'll have a hard time overeating. It's hard, but not impossible, to gain fat eating lean meats or egg whites, vegetables, moderate fat, and limited carbs. However, if you throw carbs in the mix, it gets a whole lot easier to gain fat, as they can pack a significant amount of calories into your meals without keeping you very full.

Ultimately what determines fat loss is total calories, not any one macronutrient. Carb cycling keeps your calories in check, but there is nothing magical about it. If you want to eat carbs daily, you can do this; you just need to be mindful of your total calories. When you are eating carbs with a meal, try to keep the fat on the lower end, and still stick with your lean proteins. If you find yourself gaining weight back, you may need to track again for a week or two, see where you are overeating, and adjust accordingly. You can learn to instinctively eat for your body's needs, and make daily carbohydrate intake a regular part of your diet, but it may be a little bit harder.

Working in High-Carb Days Without Gaining Fat

All of this carb cycling and nutrition planning would be good and well if life didn't get in the way. Social events will always come up, and you'll want to plan accordingly. Perhaps it's a wedding or party, and you know the snacks and drinks will be endless. Maybe it's a significant other's birthday or a vacation. It might just be that you've been craving pizza all week, and want to grab a couple of slices and a beer Friday after work.

You can absolutely eat foods you enjoy without derailing your progress. It just takes a little bit of planning—and budgeting, if you will. Think of your weekly calories like a bank account. If you are eating your maintenance amount each day, you won't have much extra to spare for fun purchases, or in this case, meals that you wouldn't normally eat. However, you can save your calories for that special event and still be perfectly fine. If you know that you'll be feasting on Saturday night, rather than starving yourself all day to save calories and then binge eating, you can simply eat a little less throughout the week. Maybe go for smaller portions, or skip that extra dessert or snack if you aren't hungry and don't really need it.

ESSENTIAL

This planning for indulgences assumes your main goal is to maintain your weight. However, the choice is always yours. If you know that you are going on a week-long vacation and you don't mind gaining a few pounds, which you can lose later, then by all means eat what you'd like. Your diet shouldn't control your life, so if you want to have fun and eat what you want, that's perfectly fine. This section is just meant to help if you want to avoid weight gain more than you want to eat unlimited food.

If you fall off the wagon, so to speak, and indulge in an unplanned meal that strays from your plan, your best bet is just to get back on track. Maybe eat a little less the next couple of days, or don't even worry about it—it really isn't a big deal. The worst thing you can do is try to starve yourself the next day to make up for it. Slipping on one meal, or even one day, isn't going to be a problem in the grand scheme of things, so there is no reason to beat yourself up over it. Consider this: If you eat five times per day, say three meals and two snacks, that is thirty-five feedings per week. Even if you mess up four of those, that's still an 89 percent adherence rate—more than enough to see results. Don't let yourself get down about it and then give up and blow the whole day or weekend.

How to Use the Resources in This Book

Now that you've read a bit about carb cycling, you should have a much stronger understanding of the whole fat-loss process. You know about how your body burns fat, how food affects your body, and how to figure out your maintenance food intake. You've also learned how carb cycling works, the many benefits of it, and even how to implement it. You have all the knowledge you need to set up a solid nutrition and training plan to begin your journey to a leaner, healthier, and stronger body.

Knowledge alone isn't enough, however; it takes follow-through. You can read all the diet books in the world, but that won't help you out unless you actually put what you learn into action. To make this as easy as possible for you and give you all the tools you need to get started, there are a few bonuses in this book.

Recipes

This book includes more than 200 recipes for you to try. All sorts of foods are included, broken down into various categories. Nutrition information is included with the recipes, but recipe results are likely to vary from person to person, so it's best to calculate that yourself. If you need a place to find nutritional information for food, *www.nutritionvalue.org* is a great resource. Even if you use the same ingredients as given in the book, there are so many options and brands for most food items that it's impossible to give nutrition information that will always be 100 percent accurate. Especially with whole foods that aren't mass-produced the same way each time, serving sizes and nutrition content will vary.

You should have no problems, however, with reading the recipes and deciding how to fit the ones you like into your day. The recipes are simple, without too many ingredients, so a quick read to see what goes into them should give you some clues. There are also notes with each recipe that will help you even more. As a general rule, most of the recipes will include lean protein and low to moderate fat; if carbs are included, that will be very clear. You can use recipes from any source you like and make them fit your nutrition plan, but the ones in this book will be a great starting point for you.

Sample Meal Plans

The meal plans in the book are meant to serve as an example of how you could set up your day. They were not designed by a registered dietician or nutritionist, so don't assume that by following them exactly as written, you'll see dramatic results; you still need to make sure you use these recipes to hit your individualize caloric needs. They are easy to prepare, delicious, and will help you reach your goals, but they must be fit into your macronutrient needs. Every single person is different, so your plan should be built around your lifestyle for best results. The plans in this book just show a general structure for various high-carb and low-carb days, with varying meal frequencies. You can use them as a sample of how a day might be set up.

On the subject of planning, you would definitely benefit from planning out a few days ahead of time to match your exact caloric needs. Having specific meals detailed, as you'll see in the sample plans, will let you see before the day even begins what your nutrition will look like. Rather than planning each meal as you go, which is very difficult and can be stressful, it's really best to prepare a plan and stick with it.

QUESTION

Can't I just eat different foods each day for variety?
Yes, of course, if you are okay with tracking as you go and adjusting on the fly. If you have a lot of free time, or flexibility to eat whatever you want when you want, then by all means go for variety. Just be mindful about this, as it's easy to consume all of your carbs or fat earlier in the day than planned, leaving you with limited choices for your remaining meals.

If you do stray from your plan, or want to substitute something else for a planned meal, you can quickly glance over your meals for the day and determine where to best make the change. If you have a very busy schedule or a family to take care of, planning your meals can also make shopping and meal preparations much simpler. You can choose lunches and snacks that are quick and easy and prepare them in advance on a day when you have free time.

CHAPTER 6

Breakfast

Greek Egg Scramble
70

Southwestern Omelet
71

Chocolate Banana Protein
Pancakes
71

Apple Cinnamon Oatmeal
72

Power Wrap
72

High-Protein French Toast
73

Egg White Protein Bites
74

Two-Minute Chocolate
Strawberry Protein Bowl
75

Protein Scramble Bowl
75

Low-Calorie Bacon, Egg, and
Cheese
76

Vanilla Raspberry Protein Fluff
77

Berries and Cream Parfait
78

Spinach, Red Onion, and
Mushroom Frittata
79

Huevos Rancheros
80

Simple Sweet Potato Pancakes
81

Clean Protein Power Bars
82

Homemade Scallion Hash
Brown Cakes
83

Greek Egg Scramble

This tasty recipe is high in protein with low carbs and moderate fats. It is quick, easy to make, and a delicious meal. Adjust the ingredients as needed for personal preference.

INGREDIENTS | SERVES 1

2 large whole eggs

2 large egg whites

1 cup fresh spinach

¼ cup feta cheese

¼ cup black olives (optional)

¼ teaspoon salt

⅛ teaspoon ground black pepper

High-Fat or Low-Fat?

Depending on your goals, you can adjust this recipe to have more or less fat. Use whole eggs and full-fat cheese if you want more fat, or substitute in all egg whites and low-fat cheese if you want a lower-fat meal.

1. In a medium nonstick pan coated with cooking spray, add eggs and egg whites and set over medium heat.

2. Once eggs are partially cooked, about 3–5 minutes, add the rest of the ingredients; stir until the eggs are no longer runny, and are cooked to your desired consistency.

PER SERVING: Calories: 141 | Fat: 9g | Protein: 13g | Sodium: 641mg | Fiber: 0g | Carbohydrates: 2g | Sugar: 1g

Southwestern Omelet

This recipe packs a kick, and is a great way to start your morning. Add as much hot sauce as you dare.

INGREDIENTS | SERVES 1

1 large whole egg
2 large egg whites
¼ cup shredded Mexican cheese blend
½ cup black beans, rinsed and drained
1 tablespoon fresh cilantro
½ cup salsa, or to taste
Dash hot sauce (optional)

1. Heat medium skillet coated with cooking spray or coconut oil over medium heat.

2. In a small bowl, mix egg and egg whites, using a fork to break up the yolk. Pour mixture in the pan and cook until it begins to set.

3. Add cheese, beans, and cilantro; cook 3 minutes, then fold over into omelet.

4. Top cooked omelet with salsa and hot sauce if desired.

PER SERVING: Calories: 389 | Fat: 20g | Protein: 32g | Sodium: 791mg | Fiber: 7g | Carbohydrates: 21g | Sugar: 4g

Chocolate Banana Protein Pancakes

This delicious dessert-style breakfast will satisfy any sweet tooth, while leaving you satisfied and full.

INGREDIENTS | SERVES 2

½ cup dry quick oats
1 medium banana, mashed
2 large egg whites
1 tablespoon chocolate chips
Sugar or artificial sweetener, to taste (optional)

The Power of Oats

Oats are a great substitution for flour and can be used in many recipes. For this and other recipes, you can use the oats as is, or blend them into powder using a food processor or blender for better mixing. This recipe can also be poured into a waffle maker.

1. In a medium bowl, combine oats, banana, egg whites, and chocolate chips.

2. Pour even portions of the mix onto a griddle or heated nonstick pan heated over medium heat.

3. When mix begins to bubble and set, roughly 2 minutes per side, flip over.

4. After removed from pan, pancake can be eaten as is or topped with whatever you like.

PER SERVING: Calories: 192 | Fat: 3g | Protein: 7g | Sodium: 57mg | Fiber: 4g | Carbohydrates: 35g | Sugar: 14g

Apple Cinnamon Oatmeal

This delicious fall treat is full of natural carbs and fiber and will keep you full and warm for a long time. It can also be made in bulk and reheated later.

INGREDIENTS | SERVES 2

4 cups water

2 cups dry oats

1 large apple, diced, peeled if desired

1 teaspoon cinnamon

2 tablespoons brown sugar, or brown sugar substitute

1. In a large pan, bring water to a boil.

2. Add dry oats and cook according to directions on the package.

3. After oats have cooked and thickened, reduce to a simmer and stir in remaining ingredients.

4. Cook 2–3 more minutes, or until apple chunks have softened.

PER SERVING: Calories: 413 | Fat: 5g | Protein: 11g | Sodium: 23mg | Fiber: 10g | Carbohydrates: 83g | Sugar: 25g

Power Wrap

This power wrap is loaded with all of your macronutrients—protein, carbs, and fat. It's a great option when you know you won't get food for a while, or simply want a satisfying higher-calorie breakfast.

INGREDIENTS | SERVES 1

2 large whole eggs

½ medium avocado, peeled, pitted, and sliced

¼ cup shredded cheese, any kind

1 strip cooked turkey bacon

1 (8") whole-wheat tortilla

1. In a medium pan over medium heat, scramble eggs to your desired consistency.

2. Place eggs, avocado slices, cheese, and bacon into the tortilla and roll it up.

PER SERVING: Calories: 446 | Fat: 29g | Protein: 25g | Sodium: 732mg | Fiber: 3g | Carbohydrates: 20g | Sugar: 2g

Why Avocado?

Avocados are a very good source of potassium and monounsaturated fat, the good kind. They can be used for much more than guacamole, as this recipe shows. If you want less fat, you can always skip the avocado.

High-Protein French Toast

This take on classic French toast is delicious and full of protein.

INGREDIENTS | SERVES 2

3 large egg whites, beaten

1 tablespoon each cinnamon and sugar

½ scoop vanilla protein powder (optional)

4 slices whole-wheat or Ezekiel bread

¼ cup sugar-free maple syrup

Protein Made Easy

This breakfast is a great way to get your carbs in the morning and it has a decent amount of protein. If you want to add more protein, you can mix protein powder into your cinnamon-sugar mix—it will work best with vanilla, cinnamon swirl, or unflavored protein powder.

1. Place beaten egg whites in a shallow bowl. Place cinnamon-sugar mixture in a separate shallow bowl; mix in protein powder if desired.

2. Dip slices of bread into egg whites, coating both sides. Then dip bread into cinnamon-sugar mixture.

3. Place coated bread onto a heated pan or skillet over medium heat. Cook 1–2 minutes each side.

4. Serve with sugar-free maple syrup and any other toppings you like.

PER SERVING: Calories: 216 | Fat: 2g | Protein: 32g | Sodium: 462mg | Fiber: 1g | Carbohydrates: 26g | Sugar: 3g

Egg White Protein Bites

These low-carb, protein-packed powerhouses can be cooked in bulk and refrigerated, and be ready to go whenever you need a breakfast on the run.

INGREDIENTS | SERVES 4

2 cups egg whites

3 slices turkey bacon, chopped, uncooked

½ cup shredded cheese, any kind

¼ teaspoon salt

⅛ teaspoon ground black pepper

Pure Protein?

These little snacks are loaded with complete protein, and can have as much or as little fat as you'd like with no carbs. You can use egg whites and turkey bacon, or mix in whole egg yolks or regular bacon if you want a little more fat and flavor with your meal.

1. Heat oven to 350°F. Spray a 12-cup muffin pan with olive oil or any other cooking spray.

2. Fill each muffin cup about ¾ full with egg whites.

3. Sprinkle bacon, cheese, salt, and pepper into the muffin cups.

4. Bake 15 minutes, or until the egg whites have solidified.

PER SERVING: Calories: 142 | Fat: 6g | Protein: 20g | Sodium: 529mg | Fiber: 0g | Carbohydrates: 1g | Sugar: 1g

Two-Minute Chocolate Strawberry Protein Bowl

This quick and easy breakfast is full of protein, micronutrients from the fruit, and antioxidants. This is a very filling and easy breakfast for those with a busy schedule.

INGREDIENTS | SERVES 1

1 cup nonfat plain Greek yogurt

1 cup fresh or frozen sliced strawberries

1–2 tablespoons dark chocolate chunks

2 tablespoons sugar-free chocolate syrup

1 scoop chocolate whey protein powder (optional)

In a medium bowl, combine all ingredients and mix. The whey protein is optional, but an easy way to get an extra 20–25 grams of protein into your daily intake.

PER SERVING: Calories: 434 | Fat: 11g | Protein: 40g | Sodium: 215mg | Fiber: 9g | Carbohydrates: 46g | Sugar: 35g

What Is the Best Greek Yogurt?

These days, there are so many options for Greek yogurt. Your best bet is to go with something unflavored, to avoid extra sugar and carbs. You can use low-fat or full-fat depending on your preference.

Protein Scramble Bowl

This recipe is a really good way to get healthy fats, complete proteins, and a whole bunch of micronutrients.

INGREDIENTS | SERVES 1

2 large whole eggs

2 large egg whites

1 cup fajita vegetable mix (frozen or freshly sliced)

1 turkey sausage link, cooked

¼ cup shredded sharp Cheddar

¼ teaspoon garlic salt

Add all ingredients to a medium skillet over medium heat. Scramble mixture until it reaches your desired consistency.

PER SERVING: Calories: 469 | Fat: 26g | Protein: 44g | Sodium: 1,439mg | Fiber: 4g | Carbohydrates: 17g | Sugar: 1g

Low-Calorie Bacon, Egg, and Cheese

This breakfast classic can easily be made using very low-calorie ingredients without sacrificing any taste. This breakfast is quick, easy, and sure to please.

INGREDIENTS | SERVES 1

1 whole-grain English muffin
1 large whole egg
¼ teaspoon salt
⅛ teaspoon ground black pepper
1 slice cooked turkey bacon
1 slice fat-free cheese

Boost Your Fiber with Breakfast

It is important to include fiber in your diet, as it helps keep your digestive system functioning. An easy way to do this is to shop for high-fiber bread and English muffins, as you can usually find these with extra fiber to keep you feeling full and keep your body healthy.

1. Slice English muffin and place in a toaster.

2. While it is toasting, cook egg in a medium skillet over medium heat to your desired consistency (over easy, over medium, etc.). Add salt and pepper.

3. Place egg, cooked bacon strip, and cheese in toasted muffin and enjoy.

PER SERVING: Calories: 308 | Fat: 13g | Protein: 24g | Sodium: 1,019mg | Fiber: 1g | Carbohydrates: 24g | Sugar: 2g

Vanilla Raspberry Protein Fluff

This delicious treat could almost be considered a dessert, but is a very filling breakfast that will keep you full and energized throughout the morning.

INGREDIENTS | SERVES 2

½ cup frozen raspberries

2 scoops vanilla protein powder (casein is recommended; whey can also work)

¼ cup unsweetened vanilla almond milk

1 (3.5-gram) packet stevia, or your sweetener of choice

1. Slightly thaw berries so they are still cold, but soft.

2. Add all ingredients to a medium bowl and stir; you should have a thick, pudding-like texture.

3. Eat as is, or mix in a power blender 5–10 minutes until mixture fluffs up.

PER SERVING: Calories: 186 | Fat: 1g | Protein: 26g | Sodium: 56mg | Fiber: 3g | Carbohydrates: 19g | Sugar: 16g

What Does Fluff Refer To?

By mixing all the ingredients in a bowl, you already have a satisfying, filling treat. However, if you have a blender available, processing this mixture for 5–10 minutes can double or even triple the volume, making this taste like fruity whipped cream.

Berries and Cream Parfait

A fun and sweet breakfast, perfect for a relaxing day. You can choose high- or low-fat ingredients and make this fit whatever your caloric goals are for the meal.

INGREDIENTS | SERVES 2

1 cup vanilla Greek yogurt
½ cup fresh blueberries
½ cup fresh blackberries
½ cup fresh raspberries
½ cup fat-free whipped cream
½ cup granola or high-fiber cereal

In a parfait glass or bowl, create layers with your ingredients for a visually pleasing meal. Or you can mix all the ingredients together in a medium bowl and enjoy.

PER SERVING: Calories: 305 | Fat: 9g | Protein: 12g | Sodium: 89mg | Fiber: 8g | Carbohydrates: 46g | Sugar: 30g

Micronutrient Powerhouse

Berries are very rich in antioxidants, which help your body to remove damaging free radicals caused by stress or exercise. Use any berries you'd like in this recipe, choosing a variety of colors to get a wider selection of nutrients.

Spinach, Red Onion, and Mushroom Frittata

A delicious combination of iron-rich spinach and antioxidant-packed red onion and mushrooms, this frittata delivers lots of tasty nutrition.

INGREDIENTS | SERVES 6

6 large whole eggs
2 tablespoons water, divided
½ cup sliced or diced red onion
1 cup sliced mushrooms
1 cup fresh spinach
1 teaspoon all-natural sea salt
1 teaspoon cracked black pepper

Bone Benefits of Spinach

While spinach has long been recognized as a nutritious green for its high content of iron and complex carbohydrates, the vitamin K content of this superfood is far more impressive. With each cup of cooked spinach comes more than 181 percent of the daily recommendation for vitamin K, which has the primary role of preventing bone loss and promoting bone strength. By inhibiting the activity of *osteoclasts* (cells that act to deteriorate bone) and providing nourishment to *osteoblasts* (cells that build bone and support their structure), spinach's heavy dose of vitamin K is an essential part of any diet in need of bone-supporting benefits.

1. Preheat oven to 350°F.

2. In a mixing bowl, thoroughly combine the eggs and 1 tablespoon of water.

3. Preheat a large, ovenproof skillet over medium heat, and spray with nonstick spray.

4. Add 1 tablespoon of water and the red onion to the skillet and sauté until slightly softened, about 2 minutes.

5. Add the mushrooms to the skillet and sauté for 2 minutes.

6. Add spinach to the skillet and sauté for 1 minute before adding the egg mixture.

7. Place entire skillet into the oven and bake for 20 minutes, or until firm to touch.

8. Season with salt and pepper.

PER SERVING: Calories: 82 | Fat: 5g | Protein: 7g | Sodium: 468mg | Fiber: 0.5g | Carbohydrates: 2g | Sugar: 1g

Huevos Rancheros

Packed with clean ingredients that all provide quality nutrition, these Huevos Rancheros are a healthier version that you can actually feel good about eating.

INGREDIENTS | SERVES 4

4 (8") whole-wheat tortillas

8 large whole eggs

1 tablespoon water

2 cups Fresh Salsa (see sidebar)

2 tablespoons chopped fresh cilantro

Fresh Salsa

In a large bowl, combine 2 large beefsteak tomatoes, chopped; 2 medium avocados, peeled and chopped; ½ large red onion, peeled and chopped; ½ large red bell pepper, chopped; ½ small jalapeño, chopped and seeded; 2 cloves garlic, crushed; ¼ cup freshly squeezed lime juice; 3 tablespoons chopped cilantro; 1 teaspoon chili powder; and ¼ cup olive oil. Cover and refrigerate 2–12 hours before serving.

1. In a large skillet prepared with nonstick spray over medium heat, warm tortillas individually, about 1–2 minutes. Quickly wrap with tinfoil to keep warm until use.

2. Spray skillet with more nonstick spray and add the eggs carefully, not breaking the yolks. Cook for about 3 minutes, or until the whites turn white.

3. Add 1 tablespoon of water and cover. Continue cooking for 3–5 minutes, until desired doneness is achieved.

4. Lay 1 tortilla on each of four plates; top with 2 eggs each.

5. Return skillet to heat and add salsa to skillet, stirring constantly for 1–2 minutes or until heated through.

6. Top each tortilla's eggs with ½ cup of warmed salsa, and garnish with chopped cilantro.

PER SERVING: Calories: 271 | Fat: 12g | Protein: 17g | Sodium: 1,108mg | Fiber: 3g | Carbohydrates: 24g | Sugar: 5g

Simple Sweet Potato Pancakes

Sweet, fluffy, and packed with clean complex carbohydrates, this brightly colored breakfast option is quick, easy, nutritious, and delicious!

INGREDIENTS | SERVES 10

1 cup sweet potato purée
1 cup low-fat plain Greek yogurt
1 cup unsweetened applesauce
2 large egg whites
2 large whole eggs
2 teaspoons vanilla extract
2 tablespoons Sucanat
¼ cup 100% whole-wheat flour
1 teaspoon baking powder
1 teaspoon pumpkin pie spice
1 teaspoon cinnamon
2 tablespoons agave nectar

1. Coat a large nonstick skillet with olive oil cooking spray and place over medium heat.

2. In a large bowl, combine all ingredients except the agave nectar and mix well.

3. Scoop the batter onto the preheated skillet, using approximately ½ cup of batter per pancake.

4. Cook 2–3 minutes on each side, or until golden brown. Remove from heat, plate, and drizzle all pancakes with the agave nectar.

PER SERVING: Calories: 78 | Fat: 1g | Protein: 7g | Sodium: 52mg | Fiber: 1g | Carbohydrates: 13g | Sugar: 6g

Clean Protein Power Bars

Rather than opting for a store-bought version, try these delicious homemade power bars for breakfast. Not only are they the perfect provision of muscle-promoting protein, there's the added benefit of a burst of delicious flavor in every bite.

INGREDIENTS | SERVES 9

4 cups rolled oats

¼ cup whole-wheat flour

¼ cup ground flaxseed

2 large whole eggs

1 cup all-natural almond butter

½ cup plain or vanilla almond milk or soymilk

2 tablespoons chopped or slivered almonds

Anti-inflammatory Benefits of Flaxseed

When it comes to great sources of omega-3 fatty acids, most people think of fish as being the best provider. Flaxseed is one of the lesser known foods that packs enough of this essential acid to greatly reduce inflammation and debilitating conditions that result. In just 2 tablespoons of flaxseeds, more than 130 percent of the recommended daily intake for omega-3s is provided. Asthma, osteoporosis, osteoarthritis, rheumatoid arthritis, and even migraines can all be improved with the daily inclusion of delicious flaxseeds in any diet.

1. Spray a 9" × 9" glass pan with olive oil spray and preheat oven to 350°F.

2. In a large bowl, combine oats, flour, flaxseed, eggs, almond butter, and almond or soymilk, and blend thoroughly.

3. Pour the mixture into the prepared pan and spread evenly. Top with chopped or slivered almonds, pressing them lightly into the top of the mixture.

4. Bake for 25–35 minutes, or until firm.

5. Allow to set for 1 hour before slicing into 9 equal squares.

PER SERVING: Calories: 382 | Fat: 26g | Protein: 8g | Sodium: 27mg | Fiber: 4.5g | Carbohydrates: 28g | Sugar: 1g

Homemade Scallion Hash Brown Cakes

Traditional fat-laden recipes of this breakfast favorite get cleaned up in this new and improved version by using heart-healthy olive oil and fresh ingredients that provide complex carbohydrates and antioxidants in every crispy cake.

INGREDIENTS | SERVES 6

3 Idaho potatoes, peeled and shredded

1 cup chopped scallions

1 large whole egg

2 tablespoons 100% whole-wheat flour

1 teaspoon garlic powder

1 tablespoon extra-virgin olive oil

1 teaspoon all-natural sea salt

½ teaspoon cracked black pepper

Better Your Brain Functioning with Better Potatoes

Because potatoes have received a bad reputation as an unhealthy starchy carbohydrate, it's important to clarify that there are benefits of including clean potato recipes in your diet. With a single potato providing a whopping 20 percent of your daily recommended vitamin B_6 intake, a meal including a baked, sautéed, steamed, or mashed potato contributes to the health of your brain's processes by focusing on the most intricate of all its parts: the cell. Promoting cell production, cell regeneration and repair, and cell functioning and communication, potatoes' provision of B_6 can help boost your brain function.

1. Spray a large skillet with olive oil spray and place over medium heat.

2. In a large mixing bowl, combine shredded potatoes, scallions, egg, flour, and garlic powder.

3. Form potato mixture into 6 even servings, and mold into dense patties.

4. Heat the olive oil in the skillet for 1 minute and swirl to evenly coat.

5. Add patties to skillet, three at a time, cooking 5–7 minutes per side or until golden brown and cooked through. Season with salt and pepper.

PER SERVING: Calories: 131 | Fat: 3g | Protein: 4g | Sodium: 412mg | Fiber: 2g | Carbohydrates: 22g | Sugar: 1.5g

CHAPTER 7

Lunch

Shrimp Stir-Fry
86

Slow-Cooked Chicken
87

Turkey Burgers
88

Spaghetti Squash Crab Blend
89

Low-Fat Chicken Bacon Ranch
Sandwich
89

Sirloin Chopped Salad
90

Southwestern Fajitas
90

Spinach, Feta, and Pesto
Chicken Quesadillas
91

Tuna Salad
92

Chicken Nachos
93

Pulled Chicken BBQ Sandwich
93

Healthy Fried Rice
94

Lemon-Herb Grilled
Chicken Salad
95

Sausage and Spicy Eggs
96

Lentil Salad
97

Portobello Mushroom Salad with
Gorgonzola,
Peppers, and Bacon
98

Asparagus Salad with Hard-
Boiled Egg
99

Shrimp Stir-Fry

Cooking a big stir-fry at the beginning of the week is a really easy way to have lunches ready for the week. You can simply store the cooked food in containers in the refrigerator and reheat over the stove or in the microwave whenever you need a quick meal.

INGREDIENTS | SERVES 2

1 (16-ounce) bag frozen stir-fry vegetables

1 tablespoon olive oil

6 ounces shrimp, thawed

¼ teaspoon minced garlic

¼ teaspoon sea salt

Carb It Up

You can eat this stir-fry as is, for a protein and vegetable meal that packs a lot of nutrients. If you want to add some carbs, you can serve with rice, quinoa, pasta, or any other carb of choice. It's great as is, but also a good addition to a bowl of rice if you want a quick post-workout meal.

1. In a large pan over medium heat, cook vegetables with olive oil until thawed.

2. Add the rest of the ingredients, and cook until shrimp are fully cooked (they will turn opaque and pinkish), usually around 5 minutes.

PER SERVING: Calories: 240 | Fat: 9g | Protein: 22g | Sodium: 486mg | Fiber: 6g | Carbohydrates: 20g | Sugar: 0g

Slow-Cooked Chicken

This is the most versatile way to cook your chicken. It stays tender and moist, and it goes with anything. You can make it into a sandwich, add it to a salad or rice, or just eat it plain.

INGREDIENTS | SERVES 4

1 pound boneless, skinless chicken breast

1 (16-ounce) box low-sodium chicken broth

1 medium white onion, peeled and sliced

¼ teaspoon garlic salt

⅛ teaspoon ground black pepper

The Tastiest Chicken

Slow cooking might just be the best way to cook chicken. Baking and grilling are fine, but the chicken has a tendency to dry out when cooked with these methods. After slow-cooking, your chicken will fall apart and shred very easily, and retain a lot of its moisture. The flavor is full but not overpowering, so you can add it to other dishes or sauces without negatively impacting the flavor of the meal.

1. Trim and clean chicken and place in the bottom of slow cooker.

2. Pour in enough chicken broth to cover the top of the breast.

3. Add onion and seasonings to the slow cooker.

4. Cover slow cooker and cook on low setting 4 hours until chicken is done.

5. Remove and shred with a fork. It can be eaten immediately or saved for later use.

PER SERVING: Calories: 199 | Fat: 5g | Protein: 27g | Sodium: 914mg | Fiber: 0g | Carbohydrates: 10g | Sugar: 1g

Turkey Burgers

Turkey burgers are quick to prepare and very easy to transport. Eat them cold, reheat them, or crumble them up and add them to another meal.

INGREDIENTS | SERVES 4

1 pound ground turkey

¼ teaspoon salt

⅛ teaspoon ground black pepper

¼ cup bread crumbs

Ground Turkey—Your Secret Weapon

It can be hard to reach your protein goal. A good trick is to simply cook a bunch of ground turkey in a pan with minimal seasoning. You can store this, and then add it to pasta, eggs, burritos, or any other dish that needs a protein boost, as it's a very versatile addition without an overpowering flavor.

1. Combine all ingredients in a large bowl.

2. Mix well, then use your hands to form into 4 even burger patties.

3. Grill or cook in a skillet until burgers are cooked all the way through, about 3–4 minutes per side.

PER SERVING: Calories: 194 | Fat: 10g | Protein: 20g | Sodium: 302mg | Fiber: 0g | Carbohydrates: 5g | Sugar: 0g

Spaghetti Squash Crab Blend

This dish is very simple to make, tasty, and supplies some filling carbohydrates so you have energy for your day.

INGREDIENTS | SERVES 2

1 medium spaghetti squash

1 (6-ounce) package imitation crab meat (or 1 (6-ounce) can real lump crab meat)

½ teaspoon Old Bay seasoning, or to taste

¼ teaspoon salt

⅛ teaspoon ground black pepper

1. Preheat oven to 400°F.

2. Carefully cut squash in half lengthwise and place cut side up on a baking sheet. Bake until squash is tender, about 30–45 minutes depending on the size of the squash.

3. Peel squash away from skin with a fork and place strands in a medium bowl.

4. Add the crab meat and seasonings and mix well.

PER SERVING: Calories: 82 | Fat: 1g | Protein: 15g | Sodium: 521mg | Fiber: 1g | Carbohydrates: 3g | Sugar: 2g

Low-Fat Chicken Bacon Ranch Sandwich

Here is an awesome alternative to a chicken bacon ranch sandwich that is low-fat, delicious, and packed with protein and good carbohydrates.

INGREDIENTS | SERVES 1

2 slices whole-grain bread

3 ounces grilled chicken breast

2 slices cooked turkey bacon

2 tablespoons fat-free ranch dressing

1. Toast bread.

2. On one slice bread, layer chicken breast then bacon. Spread ranch dressing over the second slice of bread and use that piece to top the other. Serve.

PER SERVING: Calories: 442 | Fat: 390g | Protein: 37g | Sodium: 1,438mg | Fiber: 2g | Carbohydrates: 38g | Sugar: 2g

The Best Bread?

In terms of pure calories, there isn't a huge variety among various bread manufacturers. You'll likely find that most slices range from 80–140 calories. For maximum health, however, a sprouted, whole-grain bread will be full of fiber and beneficial nutrients.

Sirloin Chopped Salad

A delicious low-carb salad option that's a little more interesting than your standard grilled chicken salad and contains a variety of healthy fats to keep you full.

INGREDIENTS | SERVES 1

4 ounces cooked sirloin, sliced

2 cups mixed greens

¼ cup blue cheese crumbles

1 tablespoon chopped nuts, any kind

2 tablespoons balsamic vinaigrette, or dressing of choice

Place sirloin, greens, cheese, and nuts in a large bowl and mix to combine. Top with balsamic vinaigrette or a dressing of your choice.

PER SERVING: Calories: 568 | Fat: 38g | Protein: 46g | Sodium: 573mg | Fiber: 6g | Carbohydrates: 11g | Sugar: 3g

Southwestern Fajitas

Fajitas are a very flexible meal. Once this filling is cooked and prepared it can be reheated and eaten alone, or served with tortillas and rice for extra carbs. Serve these fajitas with shredded Mexican cheese and low-fat sour cream if desired.

INGREDIENTS | SERVES 2

6 ounces boneless, skinless chicken breast, cut into strips

1 teaspoon red pepper flakes

1 teaspoon fajita or taco seasoning

1 (16-ounce) bag mixed fajita vegetables

Dash hot sauce

1. In a medium skillet over medium heat, cook chicken, seasoned with red pepper and fajita seasoning 8–10 minutes; until chicken is no longer pink.

2. Once cooked, remove and set aside.

3. In the same skillet, add vegetables and cook 5 minutes, or until soft. Once vegetables are cooked, add chicken back to pan, add a dash of hot sauce or more to taste, and cook until heated through.

PER SERVING: Calories: 186 | Fat: 3g | Protein: 23g | Sodium: 226mg | Fiber: 6g | Carbohydrates: 19g | Sugar: 0g

Spinach, Feta, and Pesto Chicken Quesadillas

Quesadillas are very quick to throw together, especially if you use pre-made ingredients. You can cook and eat them fresh, or cook them ahead of time and reheat them later if you need to take them somewhere.

INGREDIENTS | SERVES 1

2 tablespoons pesto spread

1 (8") whole-grain tortilla or flatbread

4 ounces shredded chicken (see Slow-Cooked Chicken recipe in this chapter)

½ cup fresh baby spinach

¼ cup feta cheese

Homemade Pesto

If you have some time on your hands and want to spice things up, homemade pesto will really set this recipe off. There are plenty of recipes out there to try, but for a simple one, take fresh basil with a little minced garlic and blend in blender or food processor with a little olive oil. Adjust portions to taste.

1. Spread pesto all over tortilla and fill one half of tortilla with the chicken, spinach, and cheese.

2. Fold tortilla in half and cook in a medium nonstick pan over medium heat.

3. Flip once the bottom is golden brown, brown the other side, then serve and enjoy.

PER SERVING: Calories: 645 | Fat: 26g | Protein: 41g | Sodium: 1,404mg | Fiber: 4g | Carbohydrates: 57g | Sugar: 4g

Tuna Salad

This classic lunch can be served as a sandwich, eaten with crackers, or eaten plain. It is quick to make in large batches so you can have extra meals if you are in a rush and don't have time to cook, and it's easy to transport if you need lunch on the go.

INGREDIENTS | SERVES 1

1 (5-ounce) can tuna

2 tablespoons low-fat mayonnaise

1–2 tablespoons finely chopped celery

Dash lemon juice

¼ teaspoon salt

⅛ teaspoon ground black pepper

Place all ingredients in a medium bowl and mix to combine. Chill until ready to serve.

PER SERVING: Calories: 264 | Fat: 11g | Protein: 36g | Sodium: 1,283mg | Fiber: 0g | Carbohydrates: 3g | Sugar: 2g

Does Canned Tuna Really Have Healthy Fats?

You may see advertising on tuna cans that it is high in omega-3s, a good fat. While this is true of whole tuna, it is not always true with canned tuna. Look at the nutrition label and get tuna with higher fat if you want the omega-3s. If they advertise high omega-3s but a serving only has 0.5 gram of fat, you aren't really getting many omegas. Look for albacore tuna in water, rather than light tuna in water, if you want the omega-3s. Tuna packed in oil will usually just have higher fat due to the oil itself.

Chicken Nachos

This delicious and protein-packed snack is a great way to satisfy cravings and get a well-rounded meal containing protein, carbs, and fat.

INGREDIENTS | SERVES 1

1 serving (according to package) whole-grain tortilla chips

3 ounces shredded cooked chicken

¼ cup low-fat shredded cheese, any kind

½ cup salsa

¼ cup low-fat sour cream

1. Heat oven to 375°F.

2. Spread chips on baking pan covered with aluminum foil, and top with cooked chicken and cheese.

3. Cook 12–15 minutes. Remove and serve with salsa and sour cream.

PER SERVING: Calories: 521 | Fat: 19g | Protein: 39g | Sodium: 1,379mg | Fiber: 5g | Carbohydrates: 36g | Sugar: 7g

Pulled Chicken BBQ Sandwich

This dish is a tasty and easy way to give a zing to shredded chicken. You can use any sauce you like, including barbecue, hot wing, ranch, or whatever your favorite sauce may be.

INGREDIENTS | SERVES 1

4 ounces shredded chicken, warmed (see Slow-Cooked Chicken recipe in this chapter)

2 tablespoons barbecue sauce, or any sauce of choice

1 whole-wheat hamburger bun

1. In a medium bowl, mix warm shredded chicken and barbecue sauce, making sure to coat chicken in the sauce.

2. Place heated chicken and sauce mixture on hamburger bun and serve.

PER SERVING: Calories: 349 | Fat: 18g | Protein: 21g | Sodium: 605mg | Fiber: 1g | Carbohydrates: 24g | Sugar: 9g

Healthy Fried Rice

While not a traditional fried-rice dish, this Asian-inspired meal is quick and enjoyable. It can be eaten alone or served as a side with another dish. This is an excellent source of quick-digesting carbs for pre- or post-workout.

INGREDIENTS | SERVES 2

½ cup egg whites

1 cup cooked rice

½ cup raw mixed small vegetables (peas, carrots)

½ teaspoon soy sauce

What Rice Is the Healthiest?

It really doesn't matter what sort of rice you use. White rice, brown rice, jasmine rice, and wild rice all have very similar nutritional content. You may have heard that brown rice is healthier, but the only real difference is speed of absorption. Brown rice absorbs more slowly, but some people have issues digesting it, so it's really personal preference.

1. In a medium skillet over medium heat, cook egg whites to your desired consistency.

2. While eggs are cooking, heat rice and mixed vegetables in separate bowl in the microwave for 2 minutes.

3. Combine all ingredients in a medium bowl, adding soy sauce or other Asian sauce to your liking.

PER SERVING: Calories: 187 | Fat: 1g | Protein: 11g | Sodium: 202mg | Fiber: 3g | Carbohydrates: 35g | Sugar: 0g

Lemon-Herb Grilled Chicken Salad

This is a fresh take on grilled salad—very refreshing, and perfect for the summer when you don't want to turn your oven on. Garnish this with a slice of fresh lemon if desired.

INGREDIENTS | SERVES 1

4 ounces grilled chicken breast, sliced

1 cup mixed greens

1 tablespoon olive oil

1 tablespoon lemon juice

½ teaspoon garlic salt

¼ teaspoon rosemary

In a medium bowl, combine all the ingredients.

PER SERVING: Calories: 314 | Fat: 17g | Protein: 30g | Sodium: 146mg | Fiber: 7g | Carbohydrates: 12g | Sugar: 4g

Benefits of Lemon Juice

Lemons are very alkalizing for your body, which means they help maintain a stable pH balance. In the body, you have a certain level of acidity, called the pH balance. Too much acidity can cause fatigue, muscular cramping and pain, and shortness of breath. Lemons are also good for the liver, a very important organ in the body which acts as a detoxifying organ. Lemon is a natural cleansing agent, and it can help support the liver in its effort to detoxify your bloodstream.

Sausage and Spicy Eggs

This is a very pretty dish that is not only a delicious breakfast but is also good for lunch or a late supper. Be careful not to use too much salt; most sausage has quite a lot of salt in it, so taste first.

INGREDIENTS | SERVES 4

1 pound Italian sweet sausage

¼ cup water

1 tablespoon olive oil

2 medium red bell peppers, roasted and chopped

1 medium jalapeño, seeded and minced

8 large whole eggs

¾ cup 2% milk

2 tablespoons fresh parsley for garnish

Protein Variations

Feel free to use 1 pound of turkey sausage, regular breakfast sausage, ground beef, or even crumbled bacon instead of the Italian sausage for this recipe.

1. Cut the sausage into ¼" coins. Place them in a heavy frying pan with the water and olive oil. Bring to a boil; then turn down the heat to simmer.

2. When the sausages are brown, remove them and place on a paper towel. Add the sweet red peppers and the jalapeño to the pan, and sauté them over medium heat for 5 minutes.

3. While the peppers are sautéing, beat the eggs and milk together vigorously. Add the mixture to the pan and gently fold it over until it is puffed and moist.

4. Mix in the reserved sausage, garnish with parsley, and serve hot.

PER SERVING: Calories: 383 | Fat: 23g | Protein: 35g | Sodium: 89mg | Fiber: 2g | Carbohydrates: 8g | Sugar: 2g

Lentil Salad

This is a salad with a burst of protein. Serve it as a main lunch course or as a side.

INGREDIENTS | SERVES 4

1 (1-pound) bag lentils (green, yellow, or red)

1 medium onion, peeled and chopped

½ cup wine vinegar

½ teaspoon salt

1 medium carrot, peeled and diced

2 medium stalks celery, chopped

2 medium tomatoes, sliced

1 cup French Dressing (see sidebar)

French Dressing

In a blender, mix ⅓ cup red wine vinegar; ½ teaspoon Worcestershire sauce; 1 clove garlic, chopped; 2 tablespoons chopped fresh parsley; 1 teaspoon dried thyme; and 1 teaspoon dried rosemary. Slowly add ⅔ cup extra-virgin olive oil in a thin stream so that the ingredients will emulsify.

1. Cover the lentils with water in a medium saucepan and add the onions and wine vinegar. Bring to a boil, lower the heat, and simmer until the lentils are soft, about 45 minutes. Sprinkle with salt.

2. Toss with the diced carrot and chopped celery and then arrange the tomatoes around the mound of lentils. Sprinkle with French Dressing and serve warm or at room temperature.

PER SERVING: Calories: 287 | Fat: 20g | Protein: 7g | Sodium: 631mg | Fiber: 27g | Carbohydrates: 25g | Sugar: 6g

Portobello Mushroom Salad with Gorgonzola, Peppers, and Bacon

The hot Gorgonzola cheese sets this salad apart as an impressive lunch.

INGREDIENTS | SERVES 4

2 large portobello mushrooms

½ cup French Dressing (see sidebar recipe in this chapter)

4 strips bacon

4 ounces Gorgonzola cheese, crumbled

½ cup mayonnaise

2 cups chopped romaine lettuce

½ cup chopped roasted red pepper

Mushroom Choices

There are many varieties of mushrooms available. Brown mushrooms have a robust flavor. White button mushrooms are delicious in sauces, and the big ones work well when stuffed or grilled. Get wild mushrooms from a reputable mycologist. Never guess if a wild mushroom that you find in the woods is safe. It may be poisonous!

1. Marinate the mushrooms for 1 hour in the French Dressing. Fry the bacon in a small frying pan over medium heat until crisp; set it on paper towels and crumble it.

2. On a hot grill or in a broiler, grill the mushrooms for 3 minutes per side. Cut them into strips.

3. While the mushrooms are cooking, heat the Gorgonzola and mayonnaise in a small saucepan on low until the cheese melts.

4. Place the mushrooms on the bed of lettuce. Sprinkle with the bacon. Drizzle with the cheese mixture and garnish with roasted red peppers.

PER SERVING: Calories: 365 | Fat: 31g | Protein: 11g | Sodium: 413mg | Fiber: 12g | Carbohydrates: 12g | Sugar: 3g

Asparagus Salad with Hard-Boiled Egg

This is a lovely salad to serve during the all-too-brief asparagus season.
For an easy variation, toss in some leftover cooked or smoked salmon.

INGREDIENTS | SERVES 4

1½ pounds steamed asparagus

2 large hard-boiled eggs,
coarsely grated

3 tablespoons white wine vinegar

3 tablespoons olive oil

½ teaspoon Dijon mustard

2 tablespoons lemon juice

½ tablespoon lemon zest

2 tablespoons minced fresh dill

1 tablespoon minced Italian parsley

¼ teaspoon sea salt

1. In a large bowl, toss together the asparagus and eggs. Set aside.

2. In a small bowl, whisk together the vinegar, oil, mustard, lemon juice, lemon zest, dill, parsley, and salt. Drizzle over the asparagus and egg. Toss lightly. Serve immediately.

PER SERVING: Calories: 167 | Fat: 13g | Protein: 7g | Sodium: 194mg | Fiber: 4g | Carbohydrates: 8g | Sugar: 3g

The Perfect Hard-Boiled Egg

Place eggs in a pan with a lid. Fill the pan with cold water until it is ¾"–1" above the eggs. Bring to a full boil. Remove from heat and cover. Allow the eggs to sit 15 minutes. Drain and run under cool water. Use immediately or refrigerate.

CHAPTER 8

Dinner: Beef, Pork, and Poultry

Baked Buffalo Chicken Strips
102

Sun-Dried Tomato Stuffed
Chicken
103

Chicken and Bean Burrito
104

Papaya Pulled Pork
104

Tamarind Pot Roast
105

Mustard Pecan Chicken
106

Pesto Pork Chops
107

Argentinian Steak
108

Lean Meat Balls
109

Steakhouse Blue Cheese Burger
109

Tuscan Chicken
110

Beer Can Chicken
111

Spaghetti Marinara with Chicken
and Basil
112

Lean Turkey Meatloaf
113

Marinated Grilled Turkey Cutlets
114

Garlic-Studded Pork Roast
115

Baked Buffalo Chicken Strips

Here is a healthy and delicious alternative to the ever-popular buffalo wings. Be sure to check your wing sauce; many are low in calories, but some are made with butter, sugar, or other calorie-dense ingredients. The Homemade Buffalo Wing Sauce in Chapter 14 is a great option.

INGREDIENTS | SERVES 4

1 teaspoon ground black pepper
1 teaspoon ground cayenne pepper
½ cup flour or flour substitute
1 pound chicken tenders
½ cup buffalo wing sauce

1. Preheat oven to 450°F, and line a 13" × 9" baking pan with aluminum foil.

2. In a large bowl or zip-top bag, combine black pepper, cayenne, and flour. Add chicken tenders and toss together until chicken is covered.

3. Lay chicken tenders on prepared pan and cook 30–40 minutes or until juices run clear, flipping halfway through.

4. Remove from oven, pour buffalo sauce over tenders, and serve.

PER SERVING: Calories: 196 | Fat: 4g | Protein: 26g | Sodium: 832mg | Fiber: 1g | Carbohydrates: 13g | Sugar: 0g

Sun-Dried Tomato Stuffed Chicken

This delicious recipe is bursting with flavor. Be sure to get regular chicken breasts, not thin-sliced, so they can be cut as needed here.

INGREDIENTS | SERVES 4

1 pound boneless, skinless chicken breast

½ cup feta cheese

1 (3.5-ounce) package sun-dried tomatoes

2 tablespoons pesto

¼ teaspoon salt

¼ teaspoon pepper

1. Preheat oven to 350°F.

2. Butterfly chicken breast by slicing the long way. You want the chicken to fold open like a book, you don't want it chopped into two separate pieces.

3. Lay feta cheese, tomatoes, and pesto down one half of chicken breast. Fold chicken back over itself, using a toothpick to seal if necessary, and place in glass baking dish.

4. Season chicken with salt and pepper, and bake 35–40 minutes, or until juices run clear.

PER SERVING: Calories: 271 | Fat: 9g | Protein: 29g | Sodium: 951mg | Fiber: 3g | Carbohydrates: 12g | Sugar: 12g

Chicken and Bean Burrito

This recipe calls for cooking in a microwave, which is great for those days when you are in a rush. If you'd like, you can add low-fat sour cream to the finished burrito.

INGREDIENTS | SERVES 1

½ cup cooked pinto beans
2 teaspoons taco seasoning
2 tablespoons medium salsa
3 ounces cooked chicken
1 (8") whole-wheat tortilla
2 tablespoons low-fat cheese

1. Add pinto beans, taco seasoning, and salsa to a food processor and blend.

2. Place mixture along with the cooked chicken into tortilla, and sprinkle the cheese on top.

3. Microwave 15–25 seconds, or heat in the oven until cheese is melted.

PER SERVING: Calories: 404 | Fat: 11g | Protein: 33g | Sodium: 1,750mg | Fiber: 9g | Carbohydrates: 44g | Sugar: 5g

Papaya Pulled Pork

Papaya provides moisture, body, and flavor to this tropical pulled pork.

INGREDIENTS | SERVES 8

1 (3-pound) boneless pork shoulder roast, trimmed of fat
3 cups cubed papaya, peeled
2 tablespoons ginger juice
¼ cup pineapple juice
¼ cup tomato paste
3 serrano peppers, diced
1 medium onion, diced
5 cloves garlic, sliced
1 tablespoon yellow hot sauce
1 teaspoon sea salt
1 teaspoon chili powder
1 teaspoon paprika

1. Place all ingredients in a 4-quart slow cooker. Cook on low for 8–10 hours.

2. Remove the meat and pull apart with forks. Mash any solids in the slow cooker with a potato masher.

3. Return the meat to the slow cooker and stir to combine.

PER SERVING: Calories: 297 | Fat: 12g | Protein: 34g | Sodium: 243mg | Fiber: 2g | Carbohydrates: 11g | Sugar: 5g

Tamarind Pot Roast

Fresh tamarind pods have a fresh, bright taste that perks up any pot roast.

INGREDIENTS | SERVES 8

2½ pounds top round roast

1 teaspoon salt

1 teaspoon freshly ground black pepper

1 teaspoon paprika

1 cup flour

2 tablespoons canola oil

2 medium onions, chopped

4 cloves garlic, minced

1" knob ginger, minced

2 large carrots, sliced into coins

2 cups beef stock

4 tamarind pods, skin removed

¼ cup lemon juice

2 tablespoons dark soy sauce

Terrific Tamarind

Tamarind comes in brown, papery-looking pods with soft, edible brown pulp. It has a sour-sweet taste. It is used in a variety of candies, sauces, juices, and jams. In Ayurvedic medicine, tamarind is used to treat digestive issues.

1. Preheat oven to 350°F.

2. Season the pot roast with salt, pepper, and paprika.

3. Sprinkle the flour on a plate. Dredge the roast in the flour.

4. Heat the oil in a Dutch oven. Brown the beef on all sides. Remove to a covered dish. Add the onion, garlic, ginger, and carrots to the Dutch oven. Sauté 5 minutes.

5. Meanwhile, bring the stock and tamarind to a boil in a small saucepan, stirring frequently.

6. Add the beef back to the Dutch oven. Whisk the tamarind mixture through a strainer over the beef. Add the lemon juice and soy sauce. Bring to a boil.

7. Place Dutch oven into the oven. Cover and bake for 2½ hours.

PER SERVING: Calories: 310 | Fat: 9g | Protein: 36g | Sodium: 738mg | Fiber: 2g | Carbohydrates: 19g | Sugar: 3g

Mustard Pecan Chicken

You can use any nuts in this recipe, but pecans work especially well.

INGREDIENTS | SERVES 4

½ cup shelled pecans

2 tablespoons Dijon mustard

2 tablespoons nonfat plain Greek yogurt

4 (4-ounce) boneless, skinless chicken breasts

1 tablespoon macadamia oil

1. Place pecans in a food processor and grind until they're a medium-fine consistency.

2. In a small bowl, mix together mustard and yogurt, blending well.

3. Lay chicken breasts on a plate and spread half the mustard and yogurt mixture on one side. Sprinkle half the ground pecans over mustard mixture and press lightly with the back of a spoon to help them stick.

4. Coat a large skillet with macadamia oil and place over medium-high heat. Add chicken, pecan-side down, and cook about 4 minutes. With chicken still in the pan, spread remaining mustard-yogurt mixture on the uncoated sides.

5. Sprinkle remaining pecans on top, once again pressing them in a bit with the back of a spoon.

6. Flip breasts over carefully, doing your best not to dislodge the crust.

7. Cook another 5 minutes and serve.

PER SERVING: Calories: 262 | Fat: 17g | Protein: 26g | Sodium: 222mg | Fiber: 2g | Carbohydrates: 3g | Sugar: 1g

Pesto Pork Chops

You can use the instructions in this recipe to make the pesto, or if you already have Basil Pesto from Chapter 14, you can save time and use that.

INGREDIENTS | SERVES 4

2 cloves garlic

¼ cup fresh basil leaves

¼ cup fresh parsley leaves

Zest of ½ large lemon

2 tablespoons water

1 tablespoon olive oil

¼ teaspoon salt

4 (4-ounce) pork chops, trimmed of fat

1. First make the pesto: Place garlic in food processor and pulse until chopped. Add basil, parsley, and lemon zest and pulse until chopped. Add water, olive oil, and salt, then process until almost smooth. Transfer to serving dish.

2. Add pork chops to a large skillet over medium-high heat and cook about 5 minutes per side or until cooked through. Coat the pork chops with about half of the pesto mixture as they cook, coating each side before turning.

3. Remove pork chops to a serving dish and serve with remaining pesto.

PER SERVING: Calories: 182 | Fat: 8g | Protein: 25g | Sodium: 215mg | Fiber: 0g | Carbohydrates: 1g | Sugar: 0g

Argentinian Steak

A delicious twist on a traditional sirloin that is sure to please. This dish goes well with a side salad or garlicky greens.

INGREDIENTS | SERVES 2

2 tablespoons water
½ cup chopped fresh parsley leaves
½ cup chopped fresh cilantro leaves
1 tablespoon lemon juice
1 tablespoon olive oil
¼ teaspoon salt
¼ teaspoon ground black pepper
½ teaspoon red pepper flakes
2 (4-ounce) sirloin steaks

Which Steak to Use?

Steaks will vary cut by cut, so there is no clear best steak option. If you want lower fat, generally sirloin will be a good option. If you prefer a little more fat and flavor, rib eye is a good choice.

1. Combine water, parsley, cilantro, lemon juice, oil, salt, black pepper, and red pepper in a large bowl.

2. Place steak on grill rack or skillet over medium-high heat and cook about 4 minutes per side.

3. Transfer steak to cutting board and let stand 10 minutes.

4. Thinly slice steaks across grain. Mix with parsley and cilantro mixture. Serve.

PER SERVING: Calories: 222 | Fat: 13g | Protein: 24g | Sodium: 372mg | Fiber: 1g | Carbohydrates: 2g | Sugar: 0g

Lean Meat Balls

This recipe uses lean beef, but you can also use ground turkey or chicken. These goes well served over whole-grain spaghetti and marinara sauce, or are delicious by themselves with a side of steamed green vegetables.

INGREDIENTS | SERVES 6

1 pound extra-lean ground beef

½ cup minced onion

2 large egg whites

1 large whole egg

¼ cup oat bran

2 tablespoons low-fat grated Parmesan cheese

1 teaspoon dried oregano

½ teaspoon garlic powder

2 tablespoons skim milk

¼ teaspoon salt

¼ teaspoon ground black pepper

1. Heat oven to 375°F.

2. In a large bowl, mix all ingredients together.

3. Shape into balls roughly the size of golfballs; you should have 20 meat balls total.

4. Bake 25 minutes on a 13" × 9" baking sheet.

PER SERVING: Calories: 174 | Fat: 9g | Protein: 18g | Sodium: 187mg | Fiber: 1g | Carbohydrates: 5g | Sugar: 1g

Steakhouse Blue Cheese Burger

This delicious burger can be enjoyed by itself with a side of greens or served on a hamburger bun.

INGREDIENTS | SERVES 4

1 pound lean ground beef

1 large whole egg

¼ cup bread crumbs

1 tablespoon McCormick Grill Mates Classic Steakhouse Burger Seasoning

½ cup blue cheese crumbles

1. In a large bowl, combine meat, egg, bread crumbs, and seasoning. Mix well.

2. Form into 4 evenly shaped patties. Place patties on grill (or in skillet) and cook to desired doneness, roughly 4–5 minutes per side.

3. After first flip, sprinkle blue cheese crumbles on top of the patties and allow to melt as it cooks.

PER SERVING: Calories: 257 | Fat: 12g | Protein: 30g | Sodium: 367mg | Fiber: 0g | Carbohydrates: 5g | Sugar: 1g

Tuscan Chicken

*Here is a delicious, slow-cooked chicken recipe that stores well
and can be served with a variety of side dishes.*

INGREDIENTS | SERVES 4

¼ cup chopped onion

½ medium red bell pepper, seeded and cut into strips

½ medium green bell pepper, seeded and cut into strips

1 (8-ounce) can black beans, drained

4 (4-ounce) boneless, skinless chicken breasts

2 tablespoons olive oil

1 large tomato, diced

¼ cup low-sodium chicken broth

1 tablespoon apple cider vinegar

½ teaspoon dried oregano

1 clove garlic, crushed

¼ teaspoon salt

1. Place onion, peppers, and beans in a slow cooker.

2. Place chicken on top of vegetables and beans.

3. In a medium bowl, stir together olive oil, tomato, broth, vinegar, oregano, garlic, and salt. Pour mixture over the chicken in the slow cooker.

4. Cover the slow cooker and set it to low. Cook 6–7 hours, until chicken is no longer pink, then serve.

PER SERVING: Calories: 263 | Fat: 10g | Protein: 28g | Sodium: 513mg | Fiber: 4g | Carbohydrates: 14g | Sugar: 4g

Beer Can Chicken

The beer in this chicken simply adds moisture—you won't taste it at all. If you prefer to avoid alcohol, you can use a can of Coca-Cola. The calories for both are roughly the same, and the chicken won't absorb much of it anyway, so you don't have to worry much about counting calories.

INGREDIENTS | SERVES 6

1 (4-pound) whole chicken
2 tablespoons olive oil
1 tablespoon kosher salt
1 tablespoon ground black pepper
2 tablespoons chopped fresh thyme leaves or 1 tablespoon dried thyme
1 half-full 12-ounce can beer, opened and at room temperature

1. Remove neck and giblets from cavity of chicken. Rub chicken all over with olive oil.

2. In a small bowl, combine salt, pepper, and thyme. Sprinkle mixture over chicken.

3. Make sure beer can is only half-filled with beer, with slits cut into the top of the can with a knife. Lower chicken onto the open can, so that chicken is sitting upright with the can in its cavity.

4. Place chicken on a grill, using the legs and beer can as a tripod to support the chicken and keep it stable.

5. Cover grill. Do not check chicken for at least 1 hour. After an hour, begin checking chicken every 15 minutes or so, until a meat thermometer inserted into the thickest part of the thigh reads 160°F–165°F.

6. Carefully transfer chicken to a tray or pan, let rest 10 minutes, then serve.

PER SERVING: Calories: 410 | Fat: 13g | Protein: 64g | Sodium: 1,411mg | Fiber: 0g | Carbohydrates: 2g | Sugar: 0g

Spaghetti Marinara with Chicken and Basil

This comforting dish is perfect for a high-carb day. If you're looking for a lower-carb alternative, substitute cooked spaghetti squash or zucchini noodles for the pasta.

INGREDIENTS | SERVES 6

3 tablespoons olive oil, divided

2 small yellow onions, peeled and diced

2 cloves garlic, minced

½ cup red wine

1 (28-ounce) can crushed tomatoes

3 teaspoons salt, divided

2 teaspoons freshly ground black pepper, divided

2 teaspoons dried oregano or Italian seasoning

¾ pound (12 ounces) spaghetti

1 pound chicken tenders

½ cup basil leaves, torn or left whole

½ cup freshly shredded Parmesan cheese

Versatile Marinara

This quick marinara sauce is easily adapted to suit your taste or your desired dish. Swap the red wine for beef broth for a deeper, heartier flavor and serve with meatballs. Add in diced carrot, celery, or red and green bell pepper when sautéing the onions for added flavor, nutrition, and crunch. Adding cinnamon and allspice gives the sauce a Greek flair; serve topped with crumbled feta instead of Parmesan. Sautéed or grilled shrimp and scallops make an elegant pairing with this simple sauce. Experiment and find out what you enjoy!

1. To prepare the marinara, heat 2 tablespoons olive oil in a medium skillet or small Dutch oven over medium heat. When oil is shimmering, add onions.

2. Sauté onions, stirring occasionally, until they are translucent, about 15 minutes. Be sure onions aren't charring; if they start to burn, turn the heat down. Once onions are translucent and soft, add garlic and cook until fragrant, 1–2 minutes more, stirring to make sure nothing burns.

3. Pour wine into pan and turn heat to high. Boil until wine reduces by half, scraping the brown bits from the pan to release flavor. Add tomatoes and stir to combine. Add 2 teaspoons salt, 1 teaspoon pepper, and oregano and stir. Reduce heat to low, and simmer 20 minutes.

4. While sauce is simmering, bring a large pot of water to a boil. Add spaghetti and cook until al dente, according to package directions. Drain, place back into the hot pot, and coat with 1 tablespoon oil so pasta doesn't stick.

5. Preheat a nonstick grill pan over medium-high heat. Season chicken on both sides with 1 teaspoon salt and 1 teaspoon pepper. When pan is heated, sear chicken 5 minutes, until chicken turns white and grill marks appear. Flip and grill 4–5 minutes more, or just until the internal temperature reaches 165°F.

6. To serve, divide warm spaghetti among six plates or serving bowls. Top with marinara, and nestle chicken pieces on top or on the side. Scatter basil leaves and sprinkle with cheese.

PER SERVING: Calories: 483 | Fat: 15g | Protein: 31g | Sodium: 1,728mg | Fiber: 4g | Carbohydrates: 51g | Sugar: 6g

Lean Turkey Meatloaf

This simple recipe is an excellent low-fat, high-protein option. Pair it with vegetables on your low-carb days, and serve it with a side of rice or mashed potatoes on a high-carb day.

INGREDIENTS | SERVES 4

1½ pounds lean ground turkey

¼ cup bread crumbs

1 large whole egg

½ medium onion, peeled and grated

2 tablespoons milk

½ teaspoon salt

½ teaspoon ground black pepper

2 tablespoons ketchup

1. Preheat oven to 450°F.

2. In a large bowl, combine turkey, bread crumbs, egg, onion, milk, salt, and pepper. Do not overwork. Form into a loaf and place on a baking sheet or in a 9" × 5" bread pan.

3. Brush top with ketchup, then cook 30–35 minutes before serving. Meat should reach an internal temperature of 165°F.

PER SERVING: Calories: 313 | Fat: 16g | Protein: 32g | Sodium: 607mg | Fiber: 1g | Carbohydrates: 9g | Sugar: 3g

Marinated Grilled Turkey Cutlets

If you're serving this on a high-carb day, grill some corn on the cob alongside the turkey for an easy side dish; they cook in about the same amount of time.

INGREDIENTS | SERVES 6

6 thick-cut turkey breast cutlets

1 cup light coconut milk

1 medium onion, diced

4 cloves garlic, minced

1 small Scotch bonnet pepper, minced, seeds removed

2 tablespoons canola oil

1 tablespoon Caribbean-style curry powder

1 teaspoon fresh thyme leaves

½ teaspoon ground cayenne

½ teaspoon hot paprika

¼ teaspoon freshly grated nutmeg

1 teaspoon sea salt

1. Place all ingredients in a marinating container or resealable plastic bag. Seal and shake to distribute the ingredients. Refrigerate at least 1 hour or up to 8 hours.

2. Prepare your grill according to the manufacturer's instructions. Grease the grill grate. Remove the turkey from the marinade. Discard the marinade.

3. Grill, flipping once, until fully cooked (165°F), about 10 minutes.

PER SERVING: Calories: 255 | Fat: 14g | Protein: 29g | Sodium: 455mg | Fiber: 1g | Carbohydrates: 5g | Sugar: 1g

Why Use Fresh Herbs?

Fresh herbs have more of the original nutrients intact than dried. The flavor of fresh herbs is brighter than dried herbs. Fresh herbs also add dimension of flavor to recipes.

Garlic-Studded Pork Roast

Inserting garlic into the roast not only infuses it with flavor; it keeps the meat moist as well.

INGREDIENTS | SERVES 8

1 (2-pound) pork loin
1 head garlic, peeled
1 cup basil
1 cup Italian parsley
2 tablespoons olive oil
¼ cup lemon juice
2 tablespoons lemon zest
1 teaspoon sea salt
1 teaspoon freshly ground black pepper

Garlic's Many Uses

Garlic is a fundamental ingredient in thousands of dishes around the world. Traditionally, garlic has been used to treat the common cold. It also has antibacterial activity and has been used as an antiseptic.

1. Preheat oven to 350°F.

2. Cut slits on all sides of the loin and insert a garlic clove in each one.

3. Place the basil, parsley, olive oil, lemon juice, lemon zest, salt, and pepper in a food processor. Pulse until a paste forms.

4. Rub the paste over the pork. Place in a Dutch oven and roast for 40 minutes or until the pork is fully cooked, reaching an internal temperature between 145°F (medium-rare) and 160°F (medium). Allow pork to rest 5–10 minutes before slicing and serving.

PER SERVING: Calories: 191 | Fat: 10g | Protein: 24g | Sodium: 357mg | Fiber: 0g | Carbohydrates: 2g | Sugar: 0g

CHAPTER 9

Dinner: Fish and Shellfish

Dijon Tuna
118

Lemon and Garlic Cod Fillets
122

Coconut Garlic Shrimp
118

Shrimp Scampi
122

Shrimp-Orange Kebabs
119

Crispy Parmesan Fish Sticks
123

Spinach and Feta Salmon
119

Feta and Tuna Pasta Salad
123

Salmon Burgers
120

High-Protein Tuna Melt
124

Stuffed Salmon Fillets
121

Lemon Pepper Tilapia
124

Sun-Dried Tomato Tuna
121

Shrimp Ceviche
125

Dijon Tuna

A very simple and delicious way to prepare tuna steaks. If you live near the water, you may be able to find fresh tuna steaks at a local market. Otherwise, check your local healthy foods store to find quality steaks.

INGREDIENTS | SERVES 2

2 tablespoons Dijon mustard

1 teaspoon Worcestershire sauce

1 teaspoon lemon juice

¼ teaspoon sea salt

2 (6-ounce) tuna steaks

Choose Your Fish

This recipe goes well with tuna, but you can also substitute cod, salmon, tilapia, or any other fish you have available. It will still taste delicious.

1. Preheat oven to 375°F.

2. In a medium bowl, combine the mustard, Worcestershire sauce, lemon juice, and salt. Mix well.

3. Place tuna steaks on a 13" × 9" baking sheet and pour mustard mixture over them, making sure to coat the fish.

4. Bake 15–20 minutes, or until fish flakes easily with a fork.

PER SERVING: Calories: 255 | Fat: 9g | Protein: 40g | Sodium: 566mg | Fiber: 1g | Carbohydrates: 2g | Sugar: 0g

Coconut Garlic Shrimp

This can be served as a side dish with another meal, or enjoyed as a meal all on its own, perhaps with a side salad or bowl of greens.

INGREDIENTS | SERVES 2

1 tablespoon coconut oil

2 cloves garlic, minced

2 shallots, minced

8 ounces thawed shrimp, shelled and deveined

2 tablespoons shredded coconut, raw if possible

1 tablespoon lemon juice

1 tablespoon chopped dill

1. Heat coconut oil in a medium skillet over medium heat.

2. Add garlic and shallots and sauté about 2 minutes.

3. Add shrimp and cook 3 minutes.

4. Add remaining ingredients, stir about 1 minute, and serve.

PER SERVING: Calories: 216 | Fat: 10g | Protein: 23g | Sodium: 330mg | Fiber: 1g | Carbohydrates: 7g | Sugar: 1g

Shrimp-Orange Kebabs

The citrus–soy sauce makes these shrimp kebabs sing.

INGREDIENTS | SERVES 4

1 large navel orange, halved and cut into wedges

1 large red onion, cut into wedges

1 pound large shrimp, peeled and deveined

2 tablespoons orange juice

2 tablespoons soy sauce

Skewered

Choose skewers that have one pointy end. Skewer the food directly in the center. Each piece of food on the skewer should be of similar size for even grilling.

1. Heat grill to medium. Oil the grill rack.

2. Thread the orange wedges, onion, and shrimp on 4 skewers, beginning and ending with oranges.

3. In a small bowl, whisk together the orange juice and soy sauce. Brush the sauce over the skewers.

4. Grill kebabs until the shrimp are fully cooked, about 5 minutes total.

PER SERVING: Calories: 153 | Fat: 2g | Protein: 24g | Sodium: 616mg | Fiber: 1g | Carbohydrates: 9g | Sugar: 5g

Spinach and Feta Salmon

A delicious dinner that is packed with healthy fats. You can use lower-fat options for the yogurt and cheese if you want to lower the total calories in the meal.

INGREDIENTS | SERVES 2

2 tablespoons plain Greek yogurt

¼ cup crumbled feta cheese

1 scallion, sliced crosswise

¼ cup chopped fresh spinach

1 teaspoon olive oil

2 (6-ounce) salmon fillets

1. Preheat oven to 350°F.

2. In a medium bowl, combine yogurt, cheese, scallion, spinach, and olive oil. Mix well with a fork.

3. Spread the mixture evenly over fillets.

4. Place fillets in an 8" × 8" glass baking dish and bake 15 minutes.

PER SERVING: Calories: 319 | Fat: 17g | Protein: 37g | Sodium: 294mg | Fiber: 0g | Carbohydrates: 2g | Sugar: 2g

Salmon Burgers

Canned fish is readily available at most stores, while fresh fish can sometimes be hard to come by. This recipe for salmon patties is easy to prepare and offers variety from the standard baked fish or regular burgers.

INGREDIENTS | SERVES 2

1 (8-ounce) can salmon, drained

1 large whole egg

Dash onion powder

2 tablespoons dry oats or bread crumbs

1 teaspoon olive oil

1. Mix all ingredients except the olive oil in a large bowl, mashing together with a fork. Form mixture into 2 patties.

2. Heat oil in a medium skillet over medium heat; add the patties.

3. Cook about 4 minutes per side, carefully turning with a spatula.

PER SERVING: Calories: 265 | Fat: 13g | Protein: 30g | Sodium: 439mg | Fiber: 1g | Carbohydrates: 5g | Sugar: 0g

Dietary Fats

When it comes to dietary fats, we traditionally hear about good fats and bad fats. This refers to the nutritional breakdown, as both types of fat will still have 9 calories per gram. Good fats are usually higher in omega-3s, are anti-inflammatory, and include foods like avocados, whole eggs, and fatty cuts of fish. Bad fats tend to be higher in omega-6s, can cause inflammation, and include processed and fried foods, and trans fats.

Stuffed Salmon Fillets

A tasty way to serve salmon, with slightly less fat than the Spinach and Feta Salmon recipe in this chapter.

INGREDIENTS | SERVES 2

2 (6-ounce) salmon fillets
1 large lemon, thinly sliced
1 scallion, sliced
1 tablespoon dried oregano
1 tablespoon dried thyme

Wild-Caught Salmon versus Farm Raised

While it is more pricey, wild-caught salmon is the better option if you can afford it. Wild salmon will swim in its natural environment, eating a well-rounded diet, while farm-raised salmon are often fed a limited food supply. To get a healthier fat profile, go with wild-caught when you can.

1. Preheat oven to 425°F.

2. Slice salmon horizontally about ⅔ of the way through.

3. Stuff fillets with lemon slices, scallions, oregano, and thyme.

4. Place the stuffed fillets in a 9" × 9" glass baking dish and bake 15 minutes.

PER SERVING: Calories: 255 | Fat: 10g | Protein: 34g | Sodium: 77mg | Fiber: 2g | Carbohydrates: 5g | Sugar: 1g

Sun-Dried Tomato Tuna

This dish can be eaten alone or served with chips or celery for dipping. A great meal by itself or you can share it as an appetizer.

INGREDIENTS | SERVES 1

1 tablespoon olive oil
2 tablespoons sun-dried tomatoes
½ teaspoon dried parsley
1 clove garlic, minced
¼ teaspoon salt
⅛ teaspoon ground black pepper
4 ounces canned tuna, rinsed and drained

1. Add olive oil, sun-dried tomatoes, parsley, garlic, salt, and pepper to a blender or food processor and blend until it forms a paste.

2. Place tuna in a bowl and pour the sun-dried tomato mix over top. Mix to combine. Serve as is, or warm in the oven or microwave first.

PER SERVING: Calories: 328 | Fat: 22g | Protein: 27g | Sodium: 1,135mg | Fiber: 1g | Carbohydrates: 5g | Sugar: 3g

Lemon and Garlic Cod Fillets

Here is a simple, quick, and very lean way to get some fish in your diet.
This goes well with a garlicky mixed greens dish on the side.

INGREDIENTS | SERVES 2

1 clove garlic, minced
1 tablespoon olive oil
2 (6-ounce) cod fillets
1 tablespoon lemon pepper
¼ teaspoon garlic salt
Juice from ½ fresh large lemon

1. Preheat oven to 400°F.

2. In a small bowl, mix garlic and olive oil and brush mixture over both sides of fish, and place the fish in an oiled glass 9" × 9" baking dish.

3. Sprinkle fish with lemon pepper and garlic salt. Drizzle with lemon juice.

4. Bake 10–15 minutes, or until fish flakes easily.

PER SERVING: Calories: 257 | Fat: 8g | Protein: 41g | Sodium: 420mg | Fiber: 0g | Carbohydrates: 2g | Sugar: 0g

Shrimp Scampi

This classic dish provides a tasty way to get some carbs if served with pasta,
and the shrimp are a great source of lean protein. It can be served with greens
for a low-carb option or over a bed of pasta for a higher-carb meal.

INGREDIENTS | SERVES 2

1 tablespoon butter
4 cloves garlic, minced
1 shallot, chopped
1 pound raw large shrimp, peeled and deveined
¼ teaspoon salt
⅛ teaspoon ground black pepper
2 tablespoons lemon juice
3 tablespoons white wine

1. In a large pan, heat butter over medium-high heat and sauté garlic and shallots 2 minutes.

2. Add shrimp, and sprinkle with salt and pepper. Cook 3–4 minutes.

3. Add the lemon juice and white wine; mix it all together. Cook 1–2 minutes before serving.

PER SERVING: Calories: 339 | Fat: 10g | Protein: 46g | Sodium: 635mg | Fiber: 0g | Carbohydrates: 10g | Sugar: 1g

Crispy Parmesan Fish Sticks

These delicious fish sticks provide a high-protein, low-fat meal.
Serve with your dipping sauce of choice or eat plain.

INGREDIENTS | SERVES 4

½ cup panko bread crumbs
2 tablespoons flour or flour substitute
¼ cup grated Parmesan cheese
1 tablespoon Italian seasoning
2 large egg whites
1 pound tilapia, cut into long strips

The Leanest Fish?

In general, white fish such as cod, halibut, and tilapia will be lower in fat and have fewer calories. This is good when watching calories. Higher-fat fish, such as tuna or salmon, has more calories but also more good omega-3 fatty acids. The choice is yours.

1. Preheat oven to 400°F.

2. In a shallow bowl, combine bread crumbs, flour, cheese, and seasoning. Place egg whites in a separate shallow bowl.

3. Dip fish strips into egg whites, then roll in dry mix to coat and place on a baking sheet.

4. Once all strips have been coated, bake 15 minutes and serve.

PER SERVING: Calories: 258 | Fat: 4g | Protein: 28g | Sodium: 670mg | Fiber: 2g | Carbohydrates: 25g | Sugar: 3g

Feta and Tuna Pasta Salad

This protein and carb mix is delicious when eaten fresh. It is also very
easy to transport, and can be reheated or enjoyed cold.

INGREDIENTS | SERVES 2

1 cup whole-wheat pasta
1 (5-ounce) can tuna, rinsed and drained
⅓ cup feta cheese
3 cherry tomatoes, sliced
1 tablespoon olive oil
¼ teaspoon salt
⅛ teaspoon ground black pepper

1. Cook pasta according to the directions on the box and then drain. Place pasta in a medium bowl.

2. Add tuna and feta cheese to the hot pasta, stirring until it begins to melt.

3. Add remaining ingredients, mix well, and serve.

PER SERVING: Calories: 438 | Fat: 19g | Protein: 35g | Sodium: 881mg | Fiber: 3g | Carbohydrates: 32g | Sugar: 3g

High-Protein Tuna Melt

Like a pizza, this open-face sandwich can have all kinds of toppings.
Add any ingredients you'd like to vary the recipe.

INGREDIENTS | SERVES 1

1 whole-wheat English muffin

2 tablespoons tomato sauce or pizza sauce

1 (5-ounce) can tuna, drained

¼ cup low-fat mozzarella cheese

1 teaspoon dried oregano

¼ teaspoon garlic salt

1. Slice muffin in half and spread tomato sauce on both halves.

2. Top with tuna, cheese, seasonings, and whatever other toppings you want to add.

3. Place muffin halves on a pan in the toaster oven or regular oven and broil 2–3 minutes.

PER SERVING: Calories: 412 | Fat: 8g | Protein: 52g | Sodium: 1,287mg | Fiber: 2g | Carbohydrates: 31g | Sugar: 3g

Lemon Pepper Tilapia

A very simple, mild-tasting dish that goes well with anything. Serve over rice
or pasta, or enjoy with a side of asparagus or broccoli. You can also drizzle
the fish with olive oil to add more fats to your meal if needed.

INGREDIENTS | SERVES 4

4 (4-ounce) tilapia fillets

2 tablespoons lemon juice

¼ teaspoon lemon pepper seasoning

¼ teaspoon garlic salt

1. Preheat oven to 400°F.

2. Place fish in a 9" × 9" glass baking dish, drizzle with lemon juice, and add seasonings.

3. Bake 15–20 minutes, or until fish flakes easily.

PER SERVING: Calories: 112 | Fat: 2g | Protein: 23g | Sodium: 208mg | Fiber: 0g | Carbohydrates: 1g | Sugar: 0g

Shrimp Ceviche

This versatile mixture can be served with chips as a side dish or enjoyed in larger quantities as a standalone meal.

INGREDIENTS | SERVES 2

½ pound shrimp, peeled and cooked

½ cup diced cherry tomatoes

¼ red onion, peeled and sliced

½ cup finely chopped cilantro

½ medium avocado, peeled, pitted, and chopped

¼ teaspoon salt

⅛ teaspoon ground black pepper

1 large lime

1. Add shrimp, tomatoes, onion, cilantro, avocado, salt, and pepper to a large bowl, and mix well.

2. Cut lime in half and squeeze the juices into the mix. You can also add slices of lime for extra flavor.

3. Toss the mix well, and chill until ready to serve.

PER SERVING: Calories: 222 | Fat: 9g | Protein: 25g | Sodium: 469mg | Fiber: 5g | Carbohydrates: 12g | Sugar: 2g

CHAPTER 10

Vegetarian Mains, Sides, and Salads

Vegetarian Cakes
128

High-Protein Spread
128

Banana Oatmeal
129

Quinoa Burritos
130

Spicy Peanut Tempeh Salad
131

Baked Eggplant and Bell Pepper
131

Zucchini Oven Fries
132

Lemon Quinoa
133

Fresh Corn, Pepper, and Avocado Salad
134

Southwestern Beet Slaw
135

Bean Salad with Orange Vinaigrette
136

Simple Autumn Salad
137

Vegetable-Stuffed Poblano Peppers
138

Portobello Tacos
139

Vegetarian Cakes

This is a meat-free alternative to burgers that is simple to make and tastes delicious. Serve the way you would normally enjoy regular burgers. This can be on a bun, or by itself with a side salad.

INGREDIENTS | SERVES 4

1 (15-ounce) can black beans, drained and rinsed

2 cloves garlic, minced

3 tablespoons minced onion

1 large whole egg

¼ cup oat bran or ground oats

¼ teaspoon salt

⅛ teaspoon ground black pepper

1. Blend all ingredients in a food processor or blender.

2. Form the mixture into 4 evenly shaped patties.

3. Cook in a medium skillet sprayed with cooking spray over medium heat about 4 minutes per side.

PER SERVING: Calories: 252 | Fat: 5g | Protein: 17g | Sodium: 953mg | Fiber: 13g | Carbohydrates: 41g | Sugar: 5g

High-Protein Spread

This is a perfect appetizer or side dish. Serve with crackers, chips, or vegetables for dipping.

INGREDIENTS | SERVES 2

½ cup cottage cheese

2 ounces tofu

1 tablespoon sun-dried tomatoes

½ cup spinach

Dash dried basil

Blend all ingredients in a food processor or blender, and serve.

PER SERVING: Calories: 76 | Fat: 3g | Protein: 8g | Sodium: 243mg | Fiber: 1g | Carbohydrates: 4g | Sugar: 2g

Banana Oatmeal

This take on oatmeal can be eaten with breakfast or served as a meal for lunch or dinner. It is an excellent source of carbs, protein, and fiber.

INGREDIENTS | SERVES 1

½ medium banana, mashed

½ cup dry oats

1 cup water

4 large egg whites

1 (3.5-gram) packet stevia, or other artificial sweetener

⅛ teaspoon baking powder

1. Preheat oven to 350°F.

2. In a medium bowl, combine all ingredients and mix well. Pour mixture into an ovenproof bowl sprayed with cooking spray.

3. Bake 30 minutes, then serve.

PER SERVING: Calories: 282 | Fat: 3g | Protein: 20g | Sodium: 290mg | Fiber: 6g | Carbohydrates: 45g | Sugar: 11g

Quinoa Burritos

This recipe is a great way to eat quinoa, one of the better complete protein sources available on a vegetarian diet.

INGREDIENTS | SERVES 2

4 large egg whites
½ cup cooked quinoa
½ cup black beans
¼ cup diced red onion
2 small whole-wheat tortillas
½ cup salsa
1 cup shredded lettuce
½ cup peeled, cubed avocado

1. In a medium skillet over medium heat, cook egg whites to your desired level of doneness. Remove from heat.

2. Add cooked quinoa, black beans, and onion to the egg whites and stir to combine.

3. Spread half the mixture on each tortilla.

4. Add salsa, lettuce, and avocado, then roll into burritos and serve.

PER SERVING: Calories: 371 | Fat: 10g | Protein: 19g | Sodium: 991mg | Fiber: 10g | Carbohydrates: 53g | Sugar: 6g

Quinoa, the Complete Protein

On a vegetarian diet it's very important to ensure you are getting complete protein sources, which have all the amino acids you need. Quinoa is one of the most complete protein sources in the plant world, and should be a staple in your diet.

Spicy Peanut Tempeh Salad

Here's a healthy blend that can be served over greens, eaten as a side dish, or made into a salad.

INGREDIENTS | SERVES 2

4 ounces tempeh, cut into strips
1 cup chopped kale
1 tablespoon natural peanut butter
1 tablespoon white wine vinegar
3 tablespoons water
Pinch ground cayenne pepper
Pinch garlic powder

1. In a large pan over medium heat, cook tempeh strips and kale about 3–4 minutes or until tempeh begins to look golden.

2. Add peanut butter, vinegar, water, cayenne, and garlic powder. Mix well until tempeh is coated with the mixture. Stir about 1 minute more and then serve.

PER SERVING: Calories: 181 | Fat: 11g | Protein: 14g | Sodium: 59mg | Fiber: 2g | Carbohydrates: 12g | Sugar: 1g

Baked Eggplant and Bell Pepper

Here is a great side dish to serve with your favorite vegetarian meal.

INGREDIENTS | SERVES 2

1 medium eggplant, sliced
1 medium green bell pepper, seeded and diced
2 celery stalks, sliced
2 cloves garlic, minced
1 teaspoon dried oregano
¼ teaspoon salt
⅛ teaspoon ground black pepper
¼ cup red wine vinegar

1. Preheat oven to 400°F.

2. Place eggplant, green pepper, and celery in a 13" × 9" glass dish.

3. Sprinkle with minced garlic, oregano, salt, and black pepper.

4. Pour red wine vinegar over the top.

5. Cover dish with aluminum foil and bake 30 minutes.

PER SERVING: Calories: 85 | Fat: 1g | Protein: 3g | Sodium: 336mg | Fiber: 10g | Carbohydrates: 19g | Sugar: 8g

Zucchini Oven Fries

The perfect side dish or snack for any occasion, and goes will with any main protein dish. They can also be enjoyed alone as a snack.

INGREDIENTS | SERVES 2

1 large zucchini
1 tablespoon dried oregano
1 tablespoon cumin

1. Preheat oven to 400°F.

2. Cut zucchini into ¼" × 3" sticks (about the size of standard French fries).

3. Arrange zucchini fries on nonstick baking sheet.

4. In a small bowl, combine spices and then sprinkle over the zucchini fries.

5. Place in oven and cook 15–18 minutes.

PER SERVING: Calories: 46 | Fat: 1g | Protein: 3g | Sodium: 18mg | Fiber: 3g | Carbohydrates: 7g | Sugar: 4g

Lemon Quinoa

This is a very refreshing, flavorful way to serve your quinoa. Perfectly delicious on its own, or it can be combined with tofu or mixed greens.

INGREDIENTS | SERVES 4

2 cups water
1 cup uncooked quinoa
⅓ cup finely chopped onion
1 tablespoon olive oil
1 tablespoon lemon juice
1 teaspoon lemon zest

1. Combine water and quinoa in a medium pan and bring to a boil.

2. When quinoa is boiling, turn the heat down to medium-low and add onion. Place the lid on the pot, tilting the lid to allow steam to escape, and cook until quinoa is tender and liquid is absorbed, roughly 12–15 minutes.

3. Once quinoa is cooked, stir in olive oil, lemon juice, and zest.

PER SERVING: Calories: 193 | Fat: 6g | Protein: 6g | Sodium: 7mg | Fiber: 3g | Carbohydrates: 29g | Sugar: 1g

Fresh Corn, Pepper, and Avocado Salad

The next time you make corn on the cob, set a few ears aside for this fantastic summer salad.

INGREDIENTS | SERVES 6

3 ears fresh cooked corn
1 medium red bell pepper
1 medium ripe avocado
1 jalapeño pepper, minced
1 scallion, thinly sliced
1 clove garlic, minced
Juice of 1 fresh lime
2 tablespoons olive oil
½ teaspoon freshly ground black pepper

Corn Facts

Corn is high in vitamin C, is a great source of both protein and fiber, and contains antioxidants associated with reduced risk of cardiovascular disease and hypertension. It can be eaten hot or cold, on the cob or in single kernels, and even popped. Corn grows easily in the home garden. Its sweet taste and vibrant color adds flavor, interest, and added nutrition to any meal.

1. Cut the kernels from the corn carefully, using a very sharp knife. Place in a mixing bowl.

2. Core and dice the red pepper and peel and dice the avocado. Add to the bowl, along with the jalapeño, sliced scallion (white and green parts), and minced garlic.

3. In a small bowl, whisk together the lime juice and oil. Drizzle over the salad and toss to coat. Season with freshly ground black pepper.

4. Serve immediately or cover and refrigerate until ready to serve.

PER SERVING: Calories: 135 | Fat: 9g | Protein: 2g | Sodium: 5mg | Fiber: 3g | Carbohydrates: 13g | Sugar: 2g

Southwestern Beet Slaw

This simple salad will make a beet lover out of you! Shredded beets are combined with carrots, scallions, garlic, cilantro, and a lime vinaigrette. The resulting salad is subtly sweet, spicy, and spectacular.

INGREDIENTS | SERVES 6

3 small–medium beets

3 scallions, sliced

2 medium carrots, shredded

¼ cup chopped fresh cilantro

2 cloves garlic

Juice of 2 fresh limes

1 teaspoon olive oil

½ teaspoon salt-free chili seasoning

¼ teaspoon freshly ground black pepper

Keep Your Herbs Fresh Longer

It is often difficult to make it through an entire bunch of herbs in one sitting. Keep them fresh by storing them in a glass of water in the refrigerator. Clip off the ends as needed.

1. Trim and peel the beets, then shred. Place into a mixing bowl.

2. Add the scallions, carrots, cilantro, and garlic and stir well to combine.

3. In a small bowl, add the lime juice, olive oil, chili seasoning, and black pepper and whisk well to combine. Pour dressing over the salad and toss well to coat.

4. Serve immediately or cover and refrigerate until ready to serve.

PER SERVING: Calories: 38 | Fat: 1g | Protein: 1g | Sodium: 46mg | Fiber: 2g | Carbohydrates: 7g | Sugar: 4g

Bean Salad with Orange Vinaigrette

This three-bean salad has a citrus twist, and is best suited for a high-carb day. Canned beans make this a snap to prepare; substitute 1¾ cups of each type of beans if you make them yourself.

INGREDIENTS | SERVES 6

1 (15-ounce) can no-salt-added kidney beans

1 (15-ounce) can no-salt-added garbanzo beans

1 (15-ounce) can no-salt-added pinto beans

2 shallots, chopped

1 medium carrot, shredded

1 small bell pepper, diced

1 small stalk celery, diced

¼ cup pure maple syrup

⅓ cup apple cider vinegar

2 tablespoons freshly squeezed orange juice

1 tablespoon olive oil

1 teaspoon grated orange zest

½ teaspoon freshly ground black pepper

1. Drain and rinse all the canned beans, then place in a mixing bowl.

2. Add the chopped shallot, shredded carrot, bell pepper, and celery and stir to combine.

3. Place the remaining ingredients into a small mixing bowl and whisk well. Pour the dressing over the salad and toss to coat.

4. Serve immediately or cover and refrigerate until ready to serve.

PER SERVING: Calories: 393 | Fat: 5g | Protein: 19g | Sodium: 70mg | Fiber: 16g | Carbohydrates: 69g | Sugar: 13g

Simple Autumn Salad

A tasty combination of red leaf lettuce, red onion, fruit, and walnuts in a light and tangy vinaigrette. This salad has a moderate amount of carbs, so it could fit a high- or low-carb day.

INGREDIENTS | SERVES 4

1 large head red leaf lettuce

1 pear, thinly sliced

½ small red onion, thinly sliced

½ cup dried black mission figs, chopped

⅓ cup chopped walnuts

2 tablespoons white balsamic vinegar

2 tablespoons olive oil

1 clove garlic, minced

¼ teaspoon freshly ground black pepper

1. Wash the lettuce, pat dry, then tear into bite-sized pieces. Place in a bowl with the sliced pear, onion, figs, and walnuts. Set aside.

2. In a small bowl, add the vinegar, oil, garlic, and black pepper and whisk well to combine. Pour the dressing over the salad and toss to coat. Serve immediately.

PER SERVING: Calories: 224 | Fat: 14g | Protein: 3g | Sodium: 29mg | Fiber: 5g | Carbohydrates: 25g | Sugar: 15g

Stock Up and Save

There's nothing more irritating than running out of a crucial ingredient when you're ready to cook. And this goes doubly when you're crunched for time or don't have the luxury of ordering out. By buying items in bulk, you'll not only be saving money, as per-unit costs are often cheaper, you'll also be hedging against future inconvenience.

Vegetable-Stuffed Poblano Peppers

This lean dish is best suited for a high-carb day. Large, unwrinkled poblano peppers work well in this recipe.

INGREDIENTS | SERVES 4

2 tablespoons olive oil

4 cloves garlic, minced

1 medium onion, minced

2 chipotle chilies in adobo sauce, minced

2 medium zucchini, cubed

1½ cups fresh corn kernels

¾ cup defrosted, drained chopped spinach

4 large poblano peppers

1 (28-ounce) can crushed tomatoes

1. Preheat oven to 350°F.

2. Heat oil in a skillet. Add the garlic and onion. Sauté until the onion is softened, then add the chipotle chilies, zucchini, and corn. Sauté until the zucchini begins to soften, about 5–10 minutes. Pour mixture into a bowl and stir in the spinach.

3. Slice the poblanos down the middle but not all the way through, to form a pocket. Fill each with the vegetable mixture.

4. Pour half of the tomatoes on the bottom of an 8" × 8" baking dish. Arrange the peppers open-side up in a single row. Drizzle with remaining tomatoes.

5. Bake for 20 minutes or until cooked through.

PER SERVING: Calories: 221 | Fat: 8g | Protein: 7g | Sodium: 32mg | Fiber: 8g | Carbohydrates: 36g | Sugar: 15g

Portobello Tacos

Meaty portobellos cook up quickly, making this a great weeknight meal.

INGREDIENTS | SERVES 6

8 portobello mushroom caps

1 tablespoon olive oil

6 (8") corn tortillas

1 pint cherry tomatoes, halved

1 cup chopped romaine lettuce

⅔ cup shredded red cabbage

¼ cup diced onion

1 medium avocado, sliced

½ cup sour cream

1. Brush each mushroom cap with oil. Heat a nonstick grill pan over medium heat. Grill the mushrooms until warmed through, about 3–5 minutes. Slice into ¼"-thick slices.

2. Evenly divide the mushrooms onto the tortillas. Pile the remaining ingredients on top of the mushrooms. Serve immediately.

PER SERVING: Calories: 211 | Fat: 12g | Protein: 6g | Sodium: 45mg | Fiber: 7g | Carbohydrates: 24g | Sugar: 6g

A Mushroom By Any Other Name

Agaricus bisporus when mature is the portobello mushroom. However, before it reaches that point it is alternately called cremini, baby bella, champignon, button mushroom, Italian brown, Swiss brown, or Roman mushroom. The name generally depends on the color of the cap.

CHAPTER 11

Vegan Mains, Sides, and Salads

Vegetable Stew with Cornmeal Dumplings
142

Red Beans and Rice
143

Mediterranean Chickpea Bake
144

Mini Vegetable Burgers
145

Arugula and Fennel Salad with Pomegranate
146

Apple Coleslaw
147

Root Vegetable Salad
148

Kale and Sea Vegetables with Orange-Sesame Dressing
149

Red Pepper and Fennel Salad
150

Cashew-Zucchini Soup
151

Saag Tofu
152

Red Onion and Olive Focaccia
153

Summer Vegetable Tian
154

Sweet and Spicy Brussels Sprouts
155

Garlicky Chickpeas and Spinach
156

Vegetable Stew with Cornmeal Dumplings

The naturally gluten-free cornmeal dumplings perfectly complement the fall vegetables in this hearty stew, making it a complete meal in one pot.

INGREDIENTS | SERVES 6

1 teaspoon olive oil

3 russet potatoes, peeled and diced

3 medium carrots, peeled and cut into ½" chunks

2 medium stalks celery, diced

1 medium onion, peeled and diced

2 rutabagas or turnips, peeled and diced

1 cup cauliflower florets

2 quarts low-sodium vegetable stock

1 tablespoon fresh thyme

1 tablespoon fresh parsley

⅔ cup water

2 tablespoons canola oil

½ cup cornmeal

2 teaspoons baking powder

½ teaspoon salt

1. Heat olive oil in a nonstick skillet over medium heat. Add all vegetables. Sauté until onions are soft and translucent, about 3–5 minutes. Add to a 4-quart slow cooker.

2. Add stock, thyme, and parsley. Stir. Cook 4–6 hours on high or 8 hours on low until the vegetables are fork-tender. Stir.

3. In a medium bowl, mix water, oil, cornmeal, baking powder, and salt. Drop in ¼-cup mounds in a single layer on top of the stew. Cover and cook on high 20 minutes without lifting the lid. The dumplings will look fluffy and light when fully cooked.

PER SERVING: Calories: 204 | Fat: 6g | Protein: 4g | Sodium: 436mg | Fiber: 6g | Carbohydrates: 35g | Sugar: 6g

Herbivore versus Omnivore

To make this a nonvegetarian nonvegan meal, use beef stock instead of vegetable broth and add 1 pound of diced, browned stew beef to the vegetables.

Red Beans and Rice

You can add an additional boost to the flavor of this dish by substituting spicy tomato-vegetable juice for the broth or water.

INGREDIENTS | SERVES 6

1 tablespoon olive oil

1 cup converted long-grain rice

1 (15-ounce) can red beans, drained and rinsed

1 (15-ounce) can pinto beans, drained and rinsed

½ teaspoon salt

1 teaspoon Italian seasoning

½ tablespoon dried onion flakes

1 (15-ounce) can diced tomatoes

1¼ cups gluten-free vegetable broth or water

1. Grease a 4-quart slow cooker with nonstick spray. Add oil and rice; stir to coat the rice in oil.

2. Add red beans, pinto beans, salt, Italian seasoning, onion flakes, tomatoes, and vegetable broth or water to the slow cooker. Stir to combine. Cover and cook on low 6 hours or until the rice is tender.

PER SERVING: Calories: 442 | Fat: 4g | Protein: 21g | Sodium: 422mg | Fiber: 18g | Carbohydrates: 83g | Sugar: 8g

Herbs and Spices

People often confuse herbs with spices. Herbs are green and are the leaves of plants—the only herb (in Western cooking) that is a flower is lavender. Frequently used herbs include parsley, basil, oregano, thyme, rosemary, mint, and Italian seasoning mix. Spices are roots, tubers, barks, or berries. These include pepper, cinnamon, nutmeg, allspice, cumin, turmeric, ginger, cardamom, and coriander.

Mediterranean Chickpea Bake

This flavorful dish can be enjoyed as a side dish or as a main course.

INGREDIENTS | SERVES 4

5 tablespoons olive oil

1 large onion, peeled and finely chopped

4 cloves garlic, minced

1 large tomato, chopped

2 teaspoons ground cumin

1 teaspoon paprika

2 large bunches fresh spinach, washed

2 cups cooked chickpeas

¼ teaspoon salt

¼ teaspoon pepper

1. Heat the olive oil in a medium frying pan over medium heat.

2. Fry onion and garlic 2–3 minutes, until onion starts to become translucent; then add tomato, cumin, and paprika. Continue cooking 5 minutes.

3. Add spinach and chickpeas to pan.

4. Reduce the heat and cover with a lid. Cook, stirring frequently, until spinach is wilted and chickpeas are tender. Add salt and pepper to taste.

PER SERVING: Calories: 352 | Fat: 20g | Protein: 13g | Sodium: 587mg | Fiber: 9g | Carbohydrates: 35g | Sugar: 5g

All-Natural Olive Oil Spray

To make your own olive oil spray, buy a clean spray bottle at a hardware store and fill it with olive oil. If you use a spray bottle that you have at home, make sure it has never contained anything that could leave a harmful residue. Use this spray as an alternative to nonstick sprays that don't taste like olive oil.

Mini Vegetable Burgers

These are quite good and are easy to make. On low-carb days, wrap them in romaine lettuce or cabbage leaves, or serve as-is. On higher-carb days, these are fantastic when stuffed in a pita pocket with tomatoes, lettuce, and sliced onion.

INGREDIENTS | SERVES 4

1 (13-ounce) can red kidney beans, drained and rinsed

½ cup dried gluten-free bread crumbs or crushed tortilla chips (more if beans are very wet)

½ cup chopped red onion

2 tablespoons barbecue sauce

1 large egg

1 teaspoon oregano, rosemary, thyme, basil, or sage

¼ teaspoon salt

¼ teaspoon pepper

½ cup cooked brown rice

2 tablespoons olive oil

1. Pulse all ingredients, except for rice and canola oil, in a food processor or blender. Turn into a medium bowl.

2. Add brown rice to the bean mixture.

3. Form the mixture into mini burgers. Heat oil to 300°F and fry the burgers until they are very hot.

PER SERVING: Calories: 251 | Fat: 10g | Protein: 11g | Sodium: 1,689mg | Fiber: 8g | Carbohydrates: 34g | Sugar: 4g

The Praises of Brown Rice

Unlike white rice, which is rice with its outer layers removed, brown rice has lost only the hard outer hull of the grain by the time it gets to the store. As a result, some prefer this variety to its more processed relative. Also, the fiber in brown rice may decrease your risk for colon cancer and can help lower cholesterol!

Arugula and Fennel Salad with Pomegranate

Pomegranates pack a high dose of beneficial health-promoting antioxidants. They are in peak season October through January; you can also substitute dried cranberries.

INGREDIENTS | SERVES 4

2 large navel oranges
1 large pomegranate
4 cups arugula
1 cup thinly sliced fennel
4 tablespoons olive oil
¼ teaspoon salt
¼ teaspoon pepper

Fennel Facts

Fennel, a crunchy and slightly sweet vegetable, is a popular Mediterranean ingredient. Fennel has a white or greenish-white bulb and long stalks with feathery green leaves stemming from the top. Fennel is closely related to cilantro, dill, carrots, and parsley.

1. Cut the tops and bottoms off oranges and then cut away the remaining peel. Slice each orange into 10–12 small pieces.

2. Remove seeds from the pomegranate.

3. Place arugula, orange pieces, pomegranate seeds, and fennel slices into a large bowl.

4. Coat the salad with olive oil and season with salt and pepper as desired.

PER SERVING: Calories: 224 | Fat: 15g | Protein: 3g | Sodium: 609mg | Fiber: 3g | Carbohydrates: 24g | Sugar: 15g

Apple Coleslaw

This coleslaw recipe is a refreshing, sweet alternative to traditional coleslaw with mayonnaise. Additionally, the sesame seeds give it a nice, nutty flavor.

INGREDIENTS | SERVES 4

2 cups packaged coleslaw mix
1 large unpeeled tart apple, chopped
½ cup chopped celery
½ cup chopped green bell pepper
¼ cup flaxseed oil
2 tablespoons lemon juice
1 teaspoon sesame seeds

1. In a medium bowl, combine coleslaw mix, apple, celery, and green pepper.

2. In a small bowl, whisk remaining ingredients. Pour over coleslaw mixture and toss to coat.

PER SERVING: Calories: 158 | Fat: 14g | Protein: 1g | Sodium: 20mg | Fiber: 3g | Carbohydrates: 9g | Sugar: 3g

Seeds versus Nuts

Nuts have a higher omega-6 to omega-3 ratio. Seeds, on the other hand, have a much different profile. Seeds have a lower saturated-fat content and are more easily digested by individuals with intestinal issues.

Root Vegetable Salad

This root salad has a nice texture and color. It will go well with any traditional fall or winter dish and will make your home smell like a holiday meal.

INGREDIENTS | SERVES 4

1 medium rutabaga, peeled and cubed
1 medium turnip, peeled and cubed
6 medium parsnips, peeled and cubed
3 tablespoons olive oil
1 tablespoon cinnamon
3 cloves garlic, chopped
1 tablespoon ground ginger
1 teaspoon ground black pepper

Root Vegetables

Roots are underappreciated parts of plants. These underground vegetables are incredibly delicious, and are recommended as a part of a balanced diet they are high in vitamin A and are a nice form of carbohydrate fuel, particularly after exercising.

1. Preheat oven to 400°F.

2. Place rutabaga, turnip, and parsnips in a roasting pan and drizzle with olive oil.

3. Sprinkle with cinnamon, garlic, ginger, and pepper.

4. Toss in the pan to coat and roast 40–50 minutes or until a toothpick slides easily through the vegetables.

PER SERVING: Calories: 247 | Fat: 11g | Protein: 4g | Sodium: 79mg | Fiber: 11g | Carbohydrates: 36g | Sugar: 15g

Kale and Sea Vegetables with Orange-Sesame Dressing

This salad is a great appetizer for an Asian-themed meal.

INGREDIENTS | SERVES 4

¼ cup wakame seaweed

½ cup sea lettuce

3 cups kale

½ teaspoon lemon juice

¼ cup fresh-squeezed orange juice

6 tablespoons plus 1 teaspoon sesame seeds

1 tablespoon kelp powder

Sea Vegetables

Sea vegetables are among the most nutritious and mineral-rich foods on Earth. Ocean water contains all the mineral elements known to humans. For example, both kelp and dulse, different types of seaweed, are excellent sources of iodine, which is an essential nutrient missing in most diets. Sea vegetables are dried and should be reconstituted by soaking them in water before eating.

1. Soak wakame and sea lettuce in water 30 minutes. Rinse vegetables and discard the water.

2. Remove stems from the kale. Roll kale leaves and chop into small pieces.

3. Sprinkle lemon juice onto the kale and massage it by hand to create a wilting effect.

4. Place orange juice, 6 tablespoons of sesame seeds, and kelp powder into a blender and blend until smooth.

5. Toss dressing with the kale and sea vegetables in a large bowl until well covered. Sprinkle the remaining sesame seeds on top.

PER SERVING: Calories: 90 | Fat: 5g | Protein: 4g | Sodium: 64mg | Fiber: 3g | Carbohydrates: 9g | Sugar: 2g

Red Pepper and Fennel Salad

Fennel has a fantastic licorice flavor that blends nicely with nuts. The red pepper adds a flash of color and a bit of sweetness to the mix.

INGREDIENTS | SERVES 2

⅓ cup pine nuts, toasted

3 tablespoons sesame seeds, toasted

2 tablespoons olive oil

1 medium red bell pepper, seeded and halved

6 leaves romaine lettuce, shredded

½ bulb fennel, diced

1 tablespoon walnut oil

Juice from 1 medium lime

½ teaspoon ground black pepper

Walnut Oil

Walnut oil cannot withstand high heat, so it's best to add it to food that has been cooked or is served raw, such as a salad. If you choose to cook with walnut oil, use a lower flame to avoid burning it.

1. Preheat broiler.

2. In a medium skillet, sauté pine nuts and sesame seeds in olive oil over medium heat 5 minutes.

3. Grill pepper under the broiler until the skin is blackened, and the flesh has softened slightly, about 5–8 minutes.

4. Place pepper halves in a paper bag to cool slightly. When cool enough to handle, remove the skin and slice the pepper into strips.

5. Combine red pepper slices, lettuce, and fennel in a large salad bowl.

6. Add walnut oil, lime juice, and black pepper to taste. Mix dressing well with salad. Add nut mixture and serve.

PER SERVING: Calories: 456 | Fat: 43g | Protein: 7g | Sodium: 37mg | Fiber: 6g | Carbohydrates: 17g | Sugar: 5g

Cashew-Zucchini Soup

Cashews make this soup thick and creamy and provide a serving of heart-healthy fat.

INGREDIENTS | SERVES 4

5 medium zucchini

1 large Vidalia onion, peeled and chopped

4 cloves garlic, chopped

½ teaspoon salt, plus more to taste

¼ teaspoon ground black pepper, plus more to taste

3 cups vegetable broth

½ cup raw cashews

½ teaspoon dried tarragon

Cashew Nut Butter

To save time, you may substitute cashew nut butter for the whole raw cashews. Enjoy the leftover cashew nut butter as a spread on sandwiches and as a dip for fresh fruit. Remember, nut butters are high in calories, so limit the portion size.

1. Coarsely chop zucchini.

2. Spray a large saucepan with nonstick cooking spray. Add onion to pan and cook 5 minutes, until soft and translucent. Add garlic and cook 1 minute. Stir in chopped zucchini, ½ teaspoon salt, and ¼ teaspoon ground pepper, and cook over medium heat, covered, stirring occasionally, 5 minutes.

3. Add broth and simmer 15 minutes.

4. Add cashews and tarragon. Purée soup in a blender in one to two batches. Fill the blender halfway to avoid burns from the hot liquid.

5. Return soup to pot; season with additional salt and pepper as desired.

PER SERVING: Calories: 117 | Fat: 8g | Protein: 6g | Sodium: 585mg | Fiber: 3g | Carbohydrates: 23g | Sugar: 2g

Saag Tofu

Saag is a stewed Indian dish made with greens—it's perhaps one of the most popular vegan dishes in Indian cuisine. This recipe features peppery, robust mustard greens.

INGREDIENTS | SERVES 4

2 tablespoons canola oil

1 medium onion, peeled and thinly sliced

3 cloves garlic, minced

2 green chilies, diced

2" knob ginger, finely diced

2 teaspoons black mustard seeds

½ teaspoon turmeric

2 teaspoons garam masala

½ teaspoon asafetida

½ teaspoon ground cayenne

16 ounces mustard greens, chopped

1¼ cups extra-firm tofu

½ cup water

1. Heat oil in a large skillet. Sauté onion, garlic, chilies, and ginger until onions are soft, about 5–10 minutes. Add mustard seeds and cook until they begin to pop.

2. Add remaining ingredients and cook until mustard greens wilt and tofu is warmed through, about 2–5 minutes.

PER SERVING: Calories: 131 | Fat: 8g | Protein: 4g | Sodium: 34mg | Fiber: 5g | Carbohydrates: 14g | Sugar: 5g

Types of Tofu

Tofu comes in many forms. Moisture-rich silken tofu has a texture similar to panna cotta. Firm tofu has a springy texture and is rather dense. Extra-firm tofu is even firmer and has most of the water removed.

Red Onion and Olive Focaccia

Red onions and olives perk up the flavor of this classic Italian bread.

INGREDIENTS | SERVES 12

1½ tablespoons active dry yeast
2½ cups lukewarm water, divided use
3½ cups flour
6 tablespoons olive oil, divided use
½ tablespoon kosher salt
⅓ cup sliced Spanish green olives
1 small red onion, peeled and
thinly sliced

Variations on Focaccia

Pretty much anything can top focaccia.
Some combinations include rosemary and
sea salt, onions and garlic, or spinach and
red pepper. Nonvegan versions often
include meat and a sprinkle of Parmesan at
the end of the cooking time.

1. In the bowl of a stand mixer, dissolve yeast in ½ cup lukewarm water. Allow to sit about 10 minutes.

2. Add flour, 4 tablespoons olive oil, remaining water, and salt. Use a dough hook to mix until a soft dough forms.

3. Remove dough from bowl and form into a round. Grease a 13" × 9" baking pan. Place dough in pan. Cover with a tea cloth and allow to rise 1½ hours.

4. Preheat oven to 450°F. Press dough into pan, reaching all corners. Allow to rise an additional 15 minutes.

5. Poke dough with the tip of your fingers to create dimples. Brush with remaining olive oil. Scatter olives and onion over the top of the bread.

6. Bake 15 minutes. Serve warm or at room temperature.

PER SERVING: Calories: 202 | Fat: 8g | Protein: 4g | Sodium: 329mg | Fiber: 1g | Carbohydrates: 29g | Sugar: 0g

Summer Vegetable Tian

Tian is a French vegetable dish consisting of a variety of thinly sliced vegetables forming a casserole.

INGREDIENTS | SERVES 4

2 tablespoons olive oil

3 cloves garlic, minced

1 medium onion, peeled and chopped

2 medium zucchini, sliced

2 medium yellow squash, sliced

3 pounds tomatoes, sliced

2 tablespoons minced basil

2 tablespoons minced oregano

1 tablespoon lemon zest

2 tablespoons lemon juice

½ teaspoon salt

½ teaspoon freshly ground black pepper

1. Heat oil in a large skillet. Add garlic and onion and sauté until onion is translucent, about 5–10 minutes.

2. Scrape garlic and onion mixture into a large bowl and add remaining ingredients. Stir until ingredients are evenly distributed.

3. Preheat oven to 400°F.

4. Arrange vegetables in a baking dish, alternating slices of zucchini, yellow squash, and tomatoes. Roast 30 minutes. Serve immediately.

PER SERVING: Calories: 172 | Fat: 8g | Protein: 6g | Sodium: 323mg | Fiber: 7g | Carbohydrates: 24g | Sugar: 15g

Variations on a Tian

Tians can be made with any variety of vegetables. Try using onion slices and eggplant. Or thinly sliced pieces of potato and winter squash for a winter version.

Sweet and Spicy Brussels Sprouts

Brussels sprouts get a bad rap, but you'll be yearning for more when you whip up this batch of Brussels whirled in sweet and spicy flavors.

INGREDIENTS | SERVES 2

2 cups Brussels sprouts

¾ cup chopped shallots, about 2 large

1 medium yellow apple, peeled and minced

¼ cup water

2 teaspoons organic maple syrup

½ teaspoon red pepper flakes

1 teaspoon all-natural sea salt

1 teaspoon cracked black pepper

1. In a large skillet over medium heat, combine Brussels sprouts, shallots, and apple with ¼ cup of water. Drizzle maple syrup over the skillet and sprinkle with red pepper flakes. Steam and sauté together until onions and apples are soft and Brussels sprouts are fork-tender, about 8–10 minutes.

2. Remove from heat and toss with sea salt and pepper.

PER SERVING: Calories: 138 | Fat: 1g | Protein: 5g | Sodium: 1,198mg | Fiber: 5g | Carbohydrates: 32g | Sugar: 14g

Eat Outside the Box Once a Week

When was the last time you ate Brussels sprouts? How about lima beans? Tempeh? Pinto beans? Whatever ingredient it is that makes you glance at a recipe and flip right past it, try it this week! Think of all the foods you thought you hated as a kid but absolutely love as an adult. Think outside the box, then go there once a week . . . and think of how many delicious foods you can try over the next 52 weeks!

Garlicky Chickpeas and Spinach

Delicious chickpeas are brightened up with aromatic garlic and vibrant spinach in this delightful side dish. It can accompany any vegan meal or act as an entrée all on its own.

INGREDIENTS | SERVES 4

1 tablespoon extra-virgin olive oil

2 cloves garlic, minced

2 cups cooked chickpeas

2 cups baby spinach leaves

8 ounces crumbled vegan soft cheese

1 teaspoon garlic powder

1 teaspoon all-natural sea salt

1 teaspoon cracked black pepper

The Mighty Chickpea

You can double or triple the nutritional greatness of chickpeas by pairing them with foods that add even more quality nutrition. To the complex carbohydrates and proteins found in the dense, creamy chickpea, you can add even more complex carbs, fiber, essential vitamins and minerals, and antioxidants just by adding some vegetables like spinach, tomatoes, broccoli, or a variety of other nutrient-dense foods.

1. In a large skillet heat olive oil and minced garlic over medium heat until garlic is golden and fragrant, about 1 minute. Add chickpeas and spinach, and sauté until beans are heated through and spinach is wilted, about 2–3 minutes.

2. Add vegan cheese and toss until melted.

3. Remove from heat and add garlic powder, salt, and pepper.

PER SERVING: Calories: 322 | Fat: 17g | Protein: 18g | Sodium: 760mg | Fiber: 7g | Carbohydrates: 27g | Sugar: 5g

CHAPTER 12

Pasta

Farfalle with Chicken and Pesto
158

Baked Ravioli
158

Whole-Wheat Penne with Kale
and Cannellini Beans
159

Artichoke and Olive Pasta
160

Broccoli-Basil Pesto and Pasta
161

Chicken and Broccoli Fettuccine
162

Pasta with Ricotta and Lemon
163

Shrimp Orzo Salad
163

Pepper, Onion, and
Shrimp Kebabs
164

High-Protein Spaghetti
164

Buttery Garlic Pasta
165

Buffalo Chicken Macaroni
and Cheese
165

Tricolor Penne
166

Shrimp Noodles with
Chinese Chives
167

Farfalle with Chicken and Pesto

*This dish is a very low-fat source of protein and carbs, and can be made to
fit your macros based on the ratio of chicken and pasta you use.*

INGREDIENTS | SERVES 4

8 ounces farfalle

½ pound fresh green beans,
ends trimmed

½ cup reserved pasta water

½ cup reduced-fat pesto sauce

2 cups bite-sized pieces grilled chicken

1. Cook pasta according to package directions. Drain and reserve ½ cup pasta water.

2. Place green beans in a shallow pan with enough fresh water to cover them. Cover and steam over medium heat 8 minutes. Drain.

3. Combine cooked pasta, pesto, reserved pasta water, chicken, and green beans in a large bowl and stir to combine.

PER SERVING: Calories: 308 | Fat: 10g | Protein: 27g | Sodium: 421mg | Fiber: 5g | Carbohydrates: 51g | Sugar: 6g

Baked Ravioli

Super fast and easy to make, for those days when you don't want to spend too much time cooking.

INGREDIENTS | SERVES 4

2 (9-ounce) packages chicken ravioli

2 cups chunky tomato sauce

¼ cup grated part-skim
mozzarella cheese

1. Preheat oven to 350°F. Cook pasta according to package directions, but only until ravioli float to the top of the saucepan. Drain.

2. Return pasta to pan and add tomato sauce, stirring to coat.

3. Pour pasta mixture into a 9" × 9" glass baking dish coated with nonstick cooking spray. Sprinkle with mozzarella cheese. Bake 15 minutes.

PER SERVING: Calories: 166 | Fat: 5g | Protein: 7g | Sodium: 1,155mg | Fiber: 2g | Carbohydrates: 33g | Sugar: 8g

Whole-Wheat Penne with Kale and Cannellini Beans

Another high-carb, low-fat meal. This pasta dish is very good to consume after a workout as it has extremely low levels of fat.

INGREDIENTS | SERVES 2

8 ounces whole-wheat penne

2 cloves garlic, minced

1 pound kale, chopped

¼ teaspoon salt

1 teaspoon red pepper flakes

1 (14-ounce) can cannellini beans, drained and rinsed

½ cup chicken broth or reserved pasta water

1. Cook pasta according to package directions. Drain.

2. Coat a medium skillet with nonstick cooking spray and sauté garlic 2 minutes over medium heat.

3. Add kale, salt, and red pepper and sauté about 8 more minutes, or until kale wilts and is tender.

4. Add beans to kale mixture along with broth and cooked pasta, stirring to combine. Cook for an additional 5–7 minutes or until beans reach desired level of softness, and serve.

PER SERVING: Calories: 362 | Fat: 3g | Protein: 17g | Sodium: 620mg | Fiber: 9g | Carbohydrates: 69g | Sugar: 3g

Artichoke and Olive Pasta

Olives add a briny savoriness to this rustic pasta dish.

INGREDIENTS | SERVES 4

2 tablespoons olive oil

3 cloves garlic, minced

2 shallots, minced

10 ounces frozen artichoke hearts, defrosted

1 cup halved large, oil-cured green olives

½ cup toasted fresh bread crumbs

⅓ cup grated Parmesan cheese

¼ cup chopped fresh Italian parsley

10 ounces hot cooked fresh linguine

1. In a saucepan, heat the oil over medium heat. Add the garlic and shallots and cook until fragrant, about 3–5 minutes.

2. Add the artichoke hearts and olives. Cook until the artichokes are cooked through, about 5 minutes.

3. Remove from heat and stir in the remaining ingredients. Serve immediately.

PER SERVING: Calories: 507 | Fat: 14g | Protein: 17g | Sodium: 546mg | Fiber: 8g | Carbohydrates: 82g | Sugar: 3g

Umami

Umami, the taste of savoriness, is one of the five basic tastes. Food rich in umami include cured meats, mushrooms, spinach, cheese, soy sauce, shrimp paste, pickles, and shellfish.

Broccoli-Basil Pesto and Pasta

A pleasant, veggie-packed change from your regular pesto.

INGREDIENTS | SERVES 8

3½ cups broccoli florets

3 (loose) cups fresh basil

3 cloves garlic

¼ teaspoon salt

½ teaspoon white pepper

3 tablespoons olive oil

¼ cup grated Parmesan cheese

3 tablespoons toasted pine nuts

1 tablespoon lemon juice

1 pound cooked pasta

How to Toast Pine Nuts

Bring out the best flavor of pine nuts, also known as pignoli nuts, by toasting them. Simply add them to a dry skillet and warm them over low heat. Watch the nuts closely so they don't burn.

1. Place the broccoli in a large pot of boiling water. Boil until tender, about 10–15 minutes. Use a slotted spoon to remove the broccoli into a bowl. Allow to cool briefly.

2. Place the broccoli in a blender or food processor. Add the remaining ingredients except the pasta. Pulse until smooth.

3. Pour pesto sauce over hot or cold pasta.

PER SERVING: Calories: 193 | Fat: 10g | Protein: 6g | Sodium: 120mg | Fiber: 3g | Carbohydrates: 22g | Sugar: 1g

Chicken and Broccoli Fettuccine

A staple at buffets, chicken, broccoli, and ziti is a great flavor combination. The nutritional problem arises when you consider its heavy cream sauce and white pasta. Light and satisfying, this version will leave you energized, not feeling weighed down!

INGREDIENTS | SERVES 2

2 tablespoons olive oil
1 boneless, skinless chicken breast
1 teaspoon minced garlic
1 cup broccoli florets
2 tablespoons filtered water
1½ cups cooked whole-wheat fettuccine
1 teaspoon all-natural sea salt

1. Prepare a skillet with 1 tablespoon of olive oil over medium heat.

2. Cut chicken breast into 1" pieces, and sauté for 2–3 minutes.

3. Add minced garlic, broccoli, and 1 tablespoon of water to skillet and continue sautéing for 4–5 minutes.

4. Add water as needed to prevent sticking and promote steaming.

5. Remove from heat when broccoli is slightly softened and the chicken is cooked through with juices running clear.

6. Toss the chicken and broccoli with the fettuccine and remaining tablespoon of olive oil. Season with the sea salt, and serve immediately.

PER SERVING: Calories: 369 | Fat: 16g | Protein: 19g | Sodium: 1,239mg | Fiber: 3g | Carbohydrates: 36g | Sugar: 1g

Pasta with Ricotta and Lemon

With only a few ingredients you can create a delicious dinner in a short time.
This pasta in a creamy cheese sauce is sure to satisfy your cravings!

INGREDIENTS | SERVES 4

1 (1-pound) box penne
2 tablespoons butter
1 cup fresh ricotta
Zest of 1 large lemon
¾ teaspoon kosher salt
¼ teaspoon freshly ground black pepper

1. Cook pasta according to package directions.

2. Reserve ⅓ cup of pasta cooking water. Drain pasta, then return it to the pot.

3. In a medium bowl, whisk together butter, ricotta, and reserved pasta water until a rich, creamy sauce forms.

4. Pour sauce over hot pasta. Add zest, salt, and pepper and toss.

PER SERVING: Calories: 577 | Fat: 15g | Protein: 21g | Sodium: 501mg | Fiber: 4g | Carbohydrates: 87g | Sugar: 4g

Shrimp Orzo Salad

Orzo is a small pasta shaped like a grain of rice. Its small size and delicate
texture make it a perfect fit for this light and refreshing salad.

INGREDIENTS | SERVES 2

8 ounces orzo
1 pound shrimp, cooked, tails removed
1 cup cherry tomatoes, sliced in half
2 ounces reduced-fat feta cheese
¼ cup chopped basil
1 tablespoon olive oil
1 tablespoon lemon juice
¼ teaspoon salt
¼ teaspoon ground black pepper

1. Cook pasta according to package directions. Drain and rinse under cool water.

2. Combine shrimp, tomatoes, orzo, feta, basil, olive oil, and lemon juice in a large bowl.

3. Season with salt and pepper, mix well, and serve.

PER SERVING: Calories: 461 | Fat: 11g | Protein: 57g | Sodium: 898mg | Fiber: 4g | Carbohydrates: 34g | Sugar: 4g

Pepper, Onion, and Shrimp Kebabs

Kebabs aren't just for chicken and steak. This delectable recipe makes a satisfying plate of juicy shrimp and crisp vegetables grilled and seasoned to perfection.

INGREDIENTS | SERVES 2

1 pound large shrimp, peeled and deveined

1 Vidalia onion, cut into 1" pieces

1 small green bell pepper, cut into 1" pieces

1 small red bell pepper, cut into 1" pieces

1 small yellow bell pepper, cut into 1" pieces

1 tablespoon olive oil

2 teaspoons garlic powder

1 teaspoon all-natural sea salt

1 teaspoon freshly ground black pepper

1. Heat a grill to medium heat, and prepare skewers.

2. Skewer the shrimp and vegetables in alternating order.

3. Paint the skewered shrimp and veggies lightly with the tablespoon of olive oil, and sprinkle with the spices.

4. Grill for 2–3 minutes on each side, or until shrimp is pink and completely cooked through.

PER SERVING: Calories: 367 | Fat: 11g | Protein: 48g | Sodium: 1,520mg | Fiber: 5g | Carbohydrates: 18g | Sugar: 7g

High-Protein Spaghetti

This incredibly simple recipe is packed with protein and carbs with minimal fat. This dish makes for perfect workout fuel.

INGREDIENTS | SERVES 2

2 ounces whole-wheat spaghetti

8 ounces ground turkey, browned

1 cup spaghetti sauce

2 tablespoons grated Parmesan cheese

Special Pastas

Many pasta companies offer higher-protein options, such as Barilla. Other companies may also add fiber or omega-3s to boost the nutrition value of their pasta. If you are looking to increase your intake of a specific nutrient, you may want to consider one of these enriched varieties.

1. Cook pasta in a large pot according to package directions, then drain and return to pot.

2. Add ground turkey and spaghetti sauce to pasta and mix well.

3. Sprinkle with cheese and serve.

PER SERVING: Calories: 368 | Fat: 19g | Protein: 30g | Sodium: 811mg | Fiber: 3g | Carbohydrates: 17g | Sugar: 6g

Buttery Garlic Pasta

A basic recipe that is the perfect side dish to your protein and vegetable meal. Neutral flavors make it easy to add to any meal where you want more carbs.

INGREDIENTS | SERVES 2

2 ounces dry angel hair, or other pasta of choice

1 tablespoon butter

1 clove garlic, minced

2 tablespoons shredded Parmesan cheese

Pinch dried parsley

1. Cook pasta in a large pot according to package directions, then drain and return pasta to pot.

2. Add butter, garlic, and cheese to the pot and stir to combine. Top with parsley before serving.

PER SERVING: Calories: 232 | Fat: 10g | Protein: 10g | Sodium: 258mg | Fiber: 3g | Carbohydrates: 25g | Sugar: 1g

Buffalo Chicken Macaroni and Cheese

Macaroni and cheese is not just for kids anymore. This twist on a classic dish packs a rich, tangy flavor with a kick, and is sure to please everyone in your family.

INGREDIENTS | SERVES 2

2 cups elbow macaroni noodles

1 tablespoon butter

½ cup fat-free shredded Cheddar cheese

6 ounces grilled chicken, cut into strips

½ cup Buffalo Wing Sauce or to taste (see recipe in Chapter 14)

½ cup blue cheese crumbles

1. Cook pasta in a large pot according to package directions, then drain pasta and return it to pot.

2. Stir butter and Cheddar cheese into the pasta until cheese begins to melt.

3. Top with grilled chicken and drizzle with Buffalo Wing Sauce.

4. Add blue cheese crumbles and serve.

PER SERVING: Calories: 688 | Fat: 20g | Protein: 43g | Sodium: 1,051mg | Fiber: 4g | Carbohydrates: 82g | Sugar: 4g

Tricolor Penne

This bulk cooked pasta is very easy to prepare, packed with lean protein, and easy to store and reheat for later meals.

INGREDIENTS | SERVES 4

1 (1-pound) box penne rigate

1 teaspoon salt, divided

1 tablespoon plus ¼ cup olive oil, divided

1¼ pounds boneless, skinless chicken breast, cut into chunks

¼ teaspoon freshly ground black pepper

1 cup grape tomatoes, cut in half

2 cups packed baby arugula

¼ cup grated Parmesan cheese

1 clove garlic

1. Cook pasta with a dash of salt according to package directions, reserving ¼ cup of pasta cooking water.

2. In a medium skillet, heat 1 tablespoon oil over medium-high heat until hot.

3. Add chicken and sprinkle with ¼ teaspoon salt and pepper; cook 4 minutes or until golden on both sides.

4. To same skillet add tomatoes and ⅛ teaspoon salt. Cook 3–4 minutes. Add mixture to pasta.

5. In blender, purée arugula, cheese, garlic, reserved pasta cooking water, ¼ teaspoon salt, and remaining ¼ cup oil until smooth. Add to pot and mix everything together, then serve.

PER SERVING: Calories: 763 | Fat: 24g | Protein: 47g | Sodium: 860mg | Fiber: 4g | Carbohydrates: 86g | Sugar: 4g

Shrimp Noodles with Chinese Chives

Chinese chives, occasionally labeled as garlic chives, look like chives but are flat and have a light, fresh-garlic scent.

INGREDIENTS | SERVES 4

8 ounces flat rice noodles

2 tablespoons canola oil

3 cloves garlic, minced

1 pound medium shrimp, peeled and deveined

1 tablespoon ginger juice

1 tablespoon fish sauce

1 pound Chinese chives, cut into 2" lengths

2 tablespoons dark soy sauce

Be a Wok Star

Buy a lightweight cast-iron wok for best results. Round bottom woks give you the most control over the food and flame. Use the smallest burner so the flame is concentrated on the bottom of the wok.

1. In a large bowl, soak the noodles in warm water for 15 minutes or until pliable.

2. Heat the oil in a large wok. Add the garlic and stir-fry until fragrant and just beginning to brown, about 2–5 minutes.

3. Add the shrimp, ginger juice, and fish sauce. Stir-fry until the shrimp is cooked, about 3–5 minutes. Add the chives. Stir-fry for 2 more minutes or until the chives have wilted.

4. Add the noodles and soy sauce. Stir-fry 5 additional minutes or until the noodles are soft. Serve immediately.

PER SERVING: Calories: 426 | Fat: 9g | Protein: 29g | Sodium: 721mg | Fiber: 4g | Carbohydrates: 54g | Sugar: 3g

CHAPTER 13

Soups

Corn and Black Bean Chili
170

Creamy Corn Chowder
171

Pumpkin Soup Base
172

Sweet Potato Soup
173

Sweet and Spicy Carrot Soup
174

Sweet Green Chickpea Soup
175

Spring Pea and Mint Soup
175

Creamy Cauliflower Soup
176

Butternut Squash and Apple
Fall Soup
177

Black Bean and King Oyster
Mushroom Soup
177

Slow Cooker Beef Stew
178

Chicken Ramen Soup
179

Cream of Broccoli Soup
180

Corn and Black Bean Chili

Most chili takes all day to cook, but this recipe has only a few ingredients and is ready very quickly.

INGREDIENTS | SERVES 4

1 pound lean ground beef

2 teaspoons chili powder

1 (14-ounce) package frozen corn and beans blend

1 (14-ounce) can low-sodium beef broth

1 (14-ounce) can seasoned tomato sauce

1. Combine ground beef and chili powder in a large Dutch oven. Cook 6 minutes over medium-high heat or until beef is browned, stirring to crumble. Drain and return to pan.

2. Stir in frozen corn mixture, broth, and tomato sauce; bring to a boil.

3. Cover, reduce heat, and simmer 10 minutes.

4. Uncover and simmer 5 minutes, stirring occasionally, then serve.

PER SERVING: Calories: 273 | Fat: 7g | Protein: 30g | Sodium: 922mg | Fiber: 4g | Carbohydrates: 26g | Sugar: 4g

Creamy Corn Chowder

Most people don't think of chowder as being the healthiest or most calorie-conscious of meal options, but this recipe breaks the mold. It's packed with delicious, all-natural ingredients specifically chosen for their nutrition and taste.

INGREDIENTS | SERVES 6

6 cups almond milk, divided

1 cup potatoes, peeled and chopped

1 cup carrots, chopped

4 cups kernel corn

1 teaspoon all-natural sea salt

1 cup low-fat plain Greek yogurt

1. In a large pot over medium heat, bring 3 cups of the almond milk, potatoes, and carrots to a boil. Reduce heat to low and simmer for 10 minutes.

2. Add remaining 3 cups almond milk, kernel corn, and salt, and simmer for another 5–8 minutes.

3. Remove the soup from the heat and allow to cool about 5 minutes.

4. Slowly mix in the Greek yogurt ¼ cup at a time until well blended.

PER SERVING: Calories: 116 | Fat: 0.3g | Protein: 7g | Sodium: 608mg | Fiber: 3g | Carbohydrates: 14g | Sugar: 4g

Pumpkin Soup Base

This soup is designed to be cooked in large amounts and then stored frozen for later use. Upon reheating, it is delicious as is, or you can add vegetables, nuts, or anything else you like.

INGREDIENTS | SERVES 6

4 medium onions, peeled and chopped

4 stalks celery, chopped

3 cloves garlic, minced

2 tablespoons olive oil

1 pound raw pumpkin, peeled, seeds removed, chopped

8 cups chicken stock, or more if needed

1. In a large saucepan over medium heat, cook onions, celery, and garlic with the oil until vegetables are soft, roughly 5 minutes.

2. Add pumpkin and enough stock to just reach the top of the pumpkin.

3. Bring mixture to a boil while stirring, then reduce the heat and simmer 40 minutes.

4. Blend this softened mixture in batches in a blender or food processor until smooth (being careful not to burn yourself with the hot liquid). Use right away or freeze for later use.

PER SERVING: Calories: 210 | Fat: 9g | Protein: 10g | Sodium: 483mg | Fiber: 2g | Carbohydrates: 24g | Sugar: 10g

Sweet Potato Soup

Sweet potatoes, which form the base of this robust soup, are a great carbohydrate source. Packed with fiber, vitamin C, and beta carotene, they are both tasty and very healthy.

INGREDIENTS | SERVES 8

6 large sweet potatoes, peeled and chopped

1 large onion, peeled and chopped

3 stalks celery, chopped

2 teaspoons poultry seasoning

1 quart chicken stock

2 cups skim milk

1. Add sweet potatoes, onion, and celery to a large pot with poultry seasoning.

2. Add chicken stock; if needed, top off with water until vegetables are just covered.

3. Boil until vegetables are soft and tender.

4. In a blender or food processor, blend softened vegetables until smooth. Add milk and blend to combine. Return to pot and heat through before serving.

PER SERVING: Calories: 652 | Fat: 9g | Protein: 28g | Sodium: 1,131mg | Fiber: 14g | Carbohydrates: 117g | Sugar: 41g

Sweet and Spicy Carrot Soup

Sweet carrots get even sweeter as they simmer in their own juices. Spiced up with ginger and shallots, the carrots take on a depth of flavor that makes this soup perfect for any occasion.

INGREDIENTS | SERVES 4

2 tablespoons ginger, grated

2 shallots, minced

4 cups water

1 pound baby carrots

¼ teaspoon cayenne pepper

Bigger Batches Save Time

Rather than having to pick and choose meals according to what ingredients you have (or don't have!) on hand, you can simplify your meal prep by having large batches of certain staples ready to go in your freezer. Stocks, soups, and sauces that save well can be made in large quantities, stored in glass containers, and frozen for weeks, making meal prep as simple as defrosting while at work or play.

1. In a pot over medium heat, combine the ginger and shallots with ¼ cup of the water. Sauté for 4–5 minutes, or until shallots are soft and translucent.

2. Add remaining water, carrots, and cayenne pepper to pot, and bring to a boil. Cover and reduce heat to low.

3. Simmer for 30–45 minutes or until carrots are fork-tender. Remove from heat.

4. Using an immersion blender, emulsify until desired thickness is achieved.

PER SERVING: Calories: 48 | Fat: 2g | Protein: 1g | Sodium: 88mg | Fiber: 4g | Carbohydrates: 11g | Sugar: 5g

Sweet Green Chickpea Soup

The delightful sweetness of peas explodes in every sip of this thick chickpea soup. With vibrant ingredients that provide essential nutrition, this recipe is a flavor-packed meal or snack that is perfect for a high-carb day.

INGREDIENTS | SERVES 4

4 cups water

1 cup broccoli spears, chopped

1 leek, cleaned and chopped

2 cups soaked chickpeas (24 hours or more of soaking is best)

4 cloves garlic, finely minced

2 cups spinach leaves, chopped

1 cup petite peas, fresh or frozen

1 teaspoon freshly cracked black pepper

1. In a large pot over medium heat, bring the water, broccoli, leek, chickpeas, and garlic to a boil. Reduce heat to low and simmer 15–20 minutes.

2. Add the spinach leaves, peas, and black pepper, and continue to cook for about 5 minutes. Remove from heat.

3. With an immersion blender, emulsify the ingredients until well blended and no bits remain.

PER SERVING: Calories: 395 | Fat: 6g | Protein: 21g | Sodium: 56mg | Fiber: 19g | Carbohydrates: 67g | Sugar: 12g

Spring Pea and Mint Soup

Incredibly simple and easy to make, this soup is a great low-calorie side dish.

INGREDIENTS | SERVES 4

1 cup chopped onion

2 tablespoons butter

2 cups chicken broth

¾ cup chopped mint leaves

¼ teaspoon salt

2 cups shelled fresh peas

1. In a large pot over medium heat, sauté onion in butter 5 minutes.

2. Add broth, mint, salt, and peas, and bring to a boil.

3. Cook 10–15 minutes, or until ingredients are soft.

4. Transfer mixture to a blender or food processor and blend until smooth, working in batches if necessary. Serve warm or cold.

PER SERVING: Calories: 189 | Fat: 8g | Protein: 8g | Sodium: 693mg | Fiber: 6g | Carbohydrates: 22g | Sugar: 6g

Creamy Cauliflower Soup

Cauliflower, a cruciferous vegetable, contains compounds that may prevent cancer. This version of cauliflower soup is perfect to serve to those with gluten allergies.

INGREDIENTS | SERVES 4

2 tablespoons olive oil

½ cup finely chopped onion

½ cup chopped celery

1 cup cauliflower florets

4 cups gluten-free chicken stock

1 cup shredded Cheddar cheese

¼ teaspoon salt

¼ teaspoon freshly ground black pepper

1 cup low-fat milk

1. Heat the oil in a large pot, and sauté the onion and celery until translucent, about 3–4 minutes. Add the cauliflower and chicken stock, and bring to a boil. Reduce heat, cover, and simmer for 25 minutes, stirring occasionally.

2. Purée the soup using an immersion blender, or carefully in batches in a food processor or blender until smooth.

3. Return the soup to the pot and bring the temperature to medium-low heat. Add the cheese, salt, and pepper, continue to cook and stir until the cheese is melted and well integrated.

4. Stir the milk into the soup. Add more chicken stock if the consistency is too thick.

PER SERVING: Calories: 291 | Fat: 18g | Protein: 17g | Sodium: 612mg | Fiber: 3g | Carbohydrates: 16g | Sugar: 4g

Butternut Squash and Apple Fall Soup

This five-ingredient classic fall soup is a delicious source of carbs that can stand alone or be served as a side dish.

INGREDIENTS | SERVES 6

1 medium butternut squash, peeled, seeded, and sliced

1 large Granny Smith apple, peeled, cored, and sliced

½ medium onion, peeled and sliced

1 teaspoon sea salt

¾ cup light cream

1. Add squash, apple, and onion to a large pot, add enough water to just cover them, and boil 20–30 minutes, until soft and tender.

2. Transfer mixture to a blender or food processor and blend until smooth, working in batches if necessary.

3. Return mixture to pot, add sea salt and cream, and stir to mix. Heat before serving.

PER SERVING: Calories: 100 | Fat: 6g | Protein: 1g | Sodium: 407mg | Fiber: 2g | Carbohydrates: 12g | Sugar: 5g

Black Bean and King Oyster Mushroom Soup

Look for large, meaty King Oyster mushrooms at an Asian grocery for the best selection and prices. Serve this soup in smaller quantities as a side dish if you plan to make it on a low-carb day.

INGREDIENTS | SERVES 4

2 tablespoons olive oil

1 medium onion, minced

1 shallot, minced

2 large carrots, minced

2 medium stalks celery, diced

1 bulb fennel, diced

6 King Oyster mushrooms, diced

2 (15-ounce) cans black beans, drained and rinsed

4 cups chicken or vegetable stock

1 tablespoon thyme leaves

½ tablespoon minced rosemary

1. Heat the oil in a Dutch oven. Sauté the onion, shallot, carrots, celery, fennel, and mushrooms until soft and fragrant, about 10–15 minutes.

2. Add the beans, stock, thyme, and rosemary. Stir. Cover and simmer 30 minutes before serving.

PER SERVING: Calories: 377 | Fat: 9g | Protein: 21g | Sodium: 736mg | Fiber: 20g | Carbohydrates: 60g | Sugar: 10g

Slow Cooker Beef Stew

Prep time on this recipe is quick, and then you leave it to cook all day and have a wonderful hearty meal waiting for you ready for dinner.

INGREDIENTS | SERVES 4

4 medium red potatoes, unpeeled and cut into quarters

1 pound beef stew meat

⅓ cup flour

½ teaspoon salt

¼ teaspoon ground black pepper

1 (14-ounce) can diced tomatoes, liquid included

2 cups water

3 cups frozen stir-fry vegetables

1. Add potatoes, beef, flour, salt, pepper, tomatoes, and water to the slow cooker; mix well.

2. Cook over low heat 7–8 hours, until beef and potatoes are tender.

3. Add frozen vegetables and cook another 30 minutes, then serve.

PER SERVING: Calories: 397 | Fat: 9g | Protein: 31g | Sodium: 524mg | Fiber: 7g | Carbohydrates: 49g | Sugar: 6g

Chicken Ramen Soup

Soup in under 10 minutes? You bet. This dish can be very quickly put together, and is a good use for precooked chicken. All you need is chicken, a package of ramen, and a few side ingredients to make this delectable dish.

INGREDIENTS | SERVES 4

3 cups water

1 (3-ounce) package chicken-flavored ramen noodles, seasoning package included

2 cups cooked and chopped chicken breast

2 bok choy leaves, sliced into strips

1 medium carrot, sliced

1 teaspoon sesame oil

1. Bring water to a boil in a large pot.

2. Add all remaining ingredients and simmer 3–5 minutes before serving.

PER SERVING: Calories: 206 | Fat: 7g | Protein: 23g | Sodium: 430mg | Fiber: 1g | Carbohydrates: 11g | Sugar: 1g

Cream of Broccoli Soup

The delicious texture of this creamy soup doesn't come from loads of heavy creams or canned soup, but from heart-healthy, protein-rich yogurt. Loaded with flavor and valuable nutrients, this is a scrumptious save of the fat-laden classic.

INGREDIENTS | SERVES 4

3 cups unsweetened almond milk

2 teaspoons all-natural sea salt

2 teaspoons garlic powder

1 teaspoon cracked black pepper

2 pounds broccoli florets

1 cup plain low-fat Greek yogurt, or soy yogurt

Broaden Your Definition of "Hearty"

Hearty bowls of soup don't have to be thick stews made of meat and thickly cut vegetables. By puréeing a blend of yogurt or milk with a combination of your favorite vegetables and ingredients, you can end up with a filling meal. Thick and hearty, or thinned and hearty, it's the vegetables and ingredients that make it a "hearty" helping.

1. In a large pot over medium heat, bring the almond milk, salt, garlic powder, pepper, and broccoli to a boil. Reduce heat to low and simmer about 10–12 minutes.

2. Remove from heat, and chill for 5 minutes. Using an immersion blender, emulsify the broccoli mixture until no bits remain.

3. Add yogurt, ¼ cup at a time, and continue blending with the immersion blender until well blended. Serve hot or cold.

PER SERVING: Calories: 149 | Fat: 1g | Protein: 14g | Sodium: 1,418mg | Fiber: 7g | Carbohydrates: 19g | Sugar: 6g

CHAPTER 14

Sauces, Dressings, and Rubs

Balsamic Vinaigrette
182

Sun-Dried Tomato Vinaigrette
183

Citrus Vinaigrette
183

Vanilla Pear Vinaigrette
184

Adobo Seasoning
184

Cajun Seasoning
185

Chicken Seasoning
185

Curry Seasoning
186

Spicy Memphis Seasoning
186

Oriental Seasoning
187

Basil Pesto
187

Homemade Buffalo Wing Sauce
188

Dry Rub for Ribs
189

Chicken Rub
189

Balsamic Vinaigrette

*A homemade, low-fat vinaigrette dressing that can be used to top salads,
or even to marinate meat, if made in larger quantities.*

INGREDIENTS | SERVES 2

1 tablespoon dried basil
¼ cup balsamic vinegar
⅓ cup finely chopped shallots
⅓ cup water
1 tablespoon olive oil
¼ teaspoon ground black pepper

Blend all ingredients in blender or food processor until smooth.

PER SERVING: Calories: 110 | Fat: 7g | Protein: 1g | Sodium: 12mg | Fiber: 1g | Carbohydrates: 11g | Sugar: 5g

Ingredient Profiles

When creating your meal plan, you may want to consider the various flavor profiles of your food to mix and match, and create delicious pairings. If it's not clear, pay attention to the spices used in the dish, and try to combine dishes that have similar flavor profiles. For example, Italian-style food, traditionally using ingredients such as basil, thyme, olive oil, and vinegars, would go well with side dishes using similar ingredients. It wouldn't necessarily match well with a spicy, Mexican-style side dish. Keeping these ingredient profiles in mind can make your diet more enjoyable.

Sun-Dried Tomato Vinaigrette

A mouthwatering Mediterranean-style dressing to go with your salad of choice.

INGREDIENTS | SERVES 2

⅓ cup sun-dried tomatoes
¼ cup red wine vinegar
1 tablespoon olive oil
1 clove garlic, minced

Blend all ingredients in blender or food processor until smooth.

PER SERVING: Calories: 90 | Fat: 7g | Protein: 1g | Sodium: 191mg | Fiber: 1g | Carbohydrates: 5g | Sugar: 3g

Citrus Vinaigrette

An Asian-style dressing that is good with grilled chicken salads or brushed on fish before cooking.

INGREDIENTS | SERVES 2

Juice of 1 large orange
Juice of 1 medium grapefruit
1 tablespoon lemon juice
1 tablespoon Dijon mustard
1 tablespoon olive oil
1 tablespoon soy sauce
2 teaspoons peeled and minced fresh ginger

Blend all ingredients in blender or food processor until smooth.

PER SERVING: Calories: 157 | Fat: 8g | Protein: 3g | Sodium: 540mg | Fiber: 4g | Carbohydrates: 23g | Sugar: 18g

Vanilla Pear Vinaigrette

This vinaigrette is a little higher in carbs, but it is low in fat and so delicious you'll want to splurge with it.

INGREDIENTS | SERVES 1

1 medium pear, peeled, cored, and halved
¼ cup white wine vinegar
½ cup water
1 teaspoon vanilla extract
¼ teaspoon salt
¼ teaspoon ground black pepper

Blend all ingredients in blender or food processor until smooth.

PER SERVING: Calories: 128 | Fat: 0g | Protein: 1g | Sodium: 600mg | Fiber: 6g | Carbohydrates: 29g | Sugar: 18g

Adobo Seasoning

This tasty seasoning is perfect for chicken, meat, fish, and vegetables.

INGREDIENTS | SERVES 2

4 tablespoons garlic powder
2 tablespoons dried oregano
2 teaspoons ground black pepper
1 teaspoon paprika

In a small bowl, mix all ingredients together. Store until ready to use.

PER SERVING: Calories: 72 | Fat: 0g | Protein: 3g | Sodium: 12mg | Fiber: 4g | Carbohydrates: 16g | Sugar: 1g

Why Make Homemade Seasonings?

You can buy pre-made seasonings, but learning how to mix your own can be fun, and you can create any flavor profile you choose. Experiment with various portions of the ingredients of these seasonings to find what you like. They are a great way to add flavor to your meals without affecting the caloric value.

Cajun Seasoning

Use this seasoning to add some kick to your meat or fish without adding a lot of calories.

INGREDIENTS | SERVES 2

1 tablespoon thyme

2 teaspoons garlic powder

2 teaspoons dried onion flakes

1 teaspoon cumin

1 teaspoon paprika

1 teaspoon fennel

½ teaspoon red pepper flakes

In a small bowl, mix all ingredients together. Store until ready to use.

PER SERVING: Calories: 23 | Fat: 1g | Protein: 1g | Sodium: 5mg | Fiber: 2g | Carbohydrates: 5g | Sugar: 1g

Chicken Seasoning

This is the perfect seasoning for your chicken, adding flavor without overpowering your dish. It works very well when batch-cooking chicken for later in the week.

INGREDIENTS | SERVES 2

1 teaspoon paprika

1 teaspoon onion powder

1 teaspoon garlic powder

1 teaspoon curry powder

½ teaspoon ground black pepper

In a small bowl, mix all ingredients together. Store until ready to use.

PER SERVING: Calories: 17 | Fat: 0g | Protein: 1g | Sodium: 3mg | Fiber: 1g | Carbohydrates: 4g | Sugar: 0g

Curry Seasoning

A very simple yet tasty seasoning that works well on both chicken and pork.

INGREDIENTS | SERVES 3

1 tablespoon curry powder
1 teaspoon onion powder
1 teaspoon garlic powder

In a small bowl, mix all ingredients together. Store until ready to use.

PER SERVING: Calories: 13 | Fat: 0g | Protein: 1g | Sodium: 2mg | Fiber: 1g | Carbohydrates: 3g | Sugar: 0g

Spicy Memphis Seasoning

This seasoning adds a kick to your meat, and also works well as a dry rub.

INGREDIENTS | SERVES 2

3 tablespoons paprika
1 tablespoon ground black pepper
1 teaspoon garlic powder
1 teaspoon ground cayenne pepper
1 teaspoon dried oregano
1 teaspoon dry mustard
1 teaspoon chili powder

In a small bowl, mix all ingredients together. Store until ready to use.

PER SERVING: Calories: 53 | Fat: 2g | Protein: 3g | Sodium: 49mg | Fiber: 6g | Carbohydrates: 11g | Sugar: 2g

Oriental Seasoning

Perfect for chicken and white fish this seasoning will add some Asian flavor to your meal. Meat cooked with this seasoning pairs well with the Citrus Vinaigrette recipe in this chapter.

INGREDIENTS | SERVES 1

2 tablespoons sesame seeds
1 teaspoon dried onion flakes
1 teaspoon garlic powder
1 teaspoon ground black pepper
1 teaspoon celery seed
1 teaspoon dried lemon zest
1 teaspoon dry mustard
1 teaspoon red pepper flakes

In a small bowl, mix all ingredients together. Store until ready to use.

PER SERVING: Calories: 138 | Fat: 10g | Protein: 5g | Sodium: 68mg | Fiber: 4g | Carbohydrates: 11g | Sugar: 1g

Basil Pesto

This is a versatile sauce that can be added to meat, pasta, or salads. It is perfect to make in summer when fresh basil is readily available and inexpensive (especially if you grow your own).

INGREDIENTS | SERVES 4

2 cups fresh basil leaves
2 cloves garlic
¼ cup pine nuts
¼ teaspoon salt
⅛ teaspoon ground black pepper
⅔ cup olive oil

1. Combine basil, garlic, pine nuts, salt, and pepper in a food processor, and blend until mixed well.

2. Add olive oil and stir. Serve immediately or store in refrigerator.

PER SERVING: Calories: 413 | Fat: 44g | Protein: 2g | Sodium: 159mg | Fiber: 2g | Carbohydrates: 4g | Sugar: 0g

Homemade Buffalo Wing Sauce

*This rich, spicy sauce is higher in fat, which makes it perfect to add
to grilled or baked chicken to add fat to your meal.*

INGREDIENTS | SERVES 4

½ cup unsalted butter
⅔ cup hot pepper sauce
1½ tablespoons white vinegar
½ teaspoon celery salt
¼ teaspoon Worcestershire sauce
¼ teaspoon ground cayenne pepper
¼ teaspoon ground white pepper
¼ teaspoon garlic powder

1. Melt butter in medium saucepan over medium heat.

2. Once melted, reduce heat to low and add remaining ingredients, whisking together.

3. Whisk 1–2 minutes over low heat, then remove and cool. Store in a jar in refrigerator or use immediately.

PER SERVING: Calories: 210 | Fat: 23g | Protein: 0g |
Sodium: 1,295mg | Fiber: 0g | Carbohydrates: 1g | Sugar: 1g

Dry Rub for Ribs

Dry rubs are meant to be rubbed into the meat before cooking. This simple mix goes wonderfully with pork ribs, especially if allowed to saturate into the meat for a while before cooking.

INGREDIENTS | SERVES 1

3 tablespoons brown sugar

1½ tablespoons paprika

1½ tablespoons salt

1½ tablespoons ground black pepper

1 teaspoon garlic powder

In a small bowl, mix all ingredients together. Use immediately or store until ready for the ribs.

PER SERVING: Calories: 220 | Fat: 2g | Protein: 3g | Sodium: 3,450mg | Fiber: 7g | Carbohydrates: 54g | Sugar: 41g

Chicken Rub

This is a versatile rub that works very well when applied to chicken before cooking. Goes well with most sauces after cooking.

INGREDIENTS | SERVES 4

¼ cup turbinado sugar

2 tablespoons paprika

1 tablespoon onion powder

2 tablespoons kosher salt

½ tablespoon garlic powder

½ tablespoon chili powder

1 tablespoon sage

½ teaspoon basil

½ teaspoon rosemary

¼ teaspoons ground cayenne pepper

In a small bowl, mix all ingredients together. Rub into chicken before cooking.

PER SERVING: Calories: 77 | Fat: 1g | Protein: 1g | Sodium: 1,165mg | Fiber: 2g | Carbohydrates: 18g | Sugar: 14g

CHAPTER 15

Sides

Kohlrabi and Swiss Chard
192

Butternut Squash Rice
193

Fondant Potatoes and Pearl
Onions
194

Roasted Beet Celeriac Mash
195

Spicy Roasted Spaghetti Squash
196

Pickled Asparagus
197

Farro with Rainbow Chard
198

Sage-Parmesan Polenta
199

Zucchini Boats
200

Ultimate Spinach and Mushroom
Risotto
201

Quinoa with Mixed Vegetables
202

Broccoli-Cauliflower Bake
203

Stuffed Mushrooms
204

Summer Squash Casserole
205

Kohlrabi and Swiss Chard

Crisp kohlrabi contrasts with silky Swiss chard to make this citrus-kissed dish.

INGREDIENTS | SERVES 4

2 tablespoons canola oil

1½ pounds kohlrabi, cubed

3 cloves garlic, minced

2 shallots, minced

2 bunches Swiss chard, chopped

¼ cup blood orange juice

2 tablespoons blood orange zest

1 teaspoon white pepper

1 teaspoon sea salt

¼ teaspoon celery seed

1. Heat oil in a large skillet. Add kohlrabi, garlic, and shallots and sauté until the kohlrabi is nearly fork-tender, about 8–20 minutes depending on thickness of kohlrabi.

2. Add remaining ingredients and sauté until Swiss chard is wilted, about 2–3 minutes.

PER SERVING: Calories: 164 | Fat: 7g | Protein: 5g | Sodium: 690mg | Fiber: 7g | Carbohydrates: 24g | Sugar: 6g

Why Use Shallots?

Shallots have a milder flavor than onions and a slightly garlic scent. They add a depth of flavor to many dishes either alone or in conjunction with onions.

Butternut Squash Rice

In this dish, the squash cooks with the rice, infusing the rice with its sweet flavor.

INGREDIENTS | SERVES 6

2 tablespoons grapeseed oil

3 cloves garlic, minced

2 shallots, minced

1 medium cubanelle pepper, diced

2 cups rice (long grain or jasmine would work well)

1 pound cubed butternut squash

1 tablespoon thyme leaves

½ teaspoon sea salt

½ teaspoon freshly ground black pepper

½ teaspoon smoked paprika

3 cups water

1. Heat oil in a Dutch oven. Add garlic, shallot, and pepper and sauté until shallots are soft, about 2–5 minutes.

2. Add rice and sauté 2 minutes.

3. Add remaining ingredients and bring to a boil. Reduce heat and simmer until rice is tender, about 15–30 minutes. Stir. Serve immediately.

PER SERVING: Calories: 343 | Fat: 6g | Protein: 7g | Sodium: 206mg | Fiber: 4g | Carbohydrates: 67g | Sugar: 3g

Fondant Potatoes and Pearl Onions

This twist on the classic French dish features nearly caramelized onions.

INGREDIENTS | SERVES 6

2 pounds unpeeled baby potatoes
1 pound pearl onions, peeled
1 tablespoon unsalted butter
1 tablespoon olive oil
½ teaspoon sea salt
½ teaspoon freshly ground black pepper
3 cups chicken stock
1 tablespoon Herbes de Provence

1. Arrange potatoes and onions in the bottom of a large, nonstick pan in a single layer. Add remaining ingredients. Bring to a boil.

2. Reduce heat and partially cover with a lid. Continue to boil until much of stock has evaporated, about 20 minutes. The potatoes should still be about half submerged in stock at this point.

3. Use a wooden spoon to press down on each potato, cracking the skin. Continue to cook until all of the stock has completely evaporated and the bottoms of the potatoes and onions are browned, about 10–25 minutes.

4. Flip potatoes and onions and cook the other side for about 5 minutes. Use a large, flat spatula to remove the potatoes and onions from the pan.

PER SERVING: Calories: 183 | Fat: 6g | Protein: 6g | Sodium: 377mg | Fiber: 4g | Carbohydrates: 28g | Sugar: 4g

Roasted Beet Celeriac Mash

Roasting beets deepens their flavors and seems to sweeten them.

INGREDIENTS | SERVES 6

4 medium beets, peeled and cubed

2 pounds celeriac, cubed

¼ cup balsamic vinegar

⅓ cup plain Greek yogurt

1 tablespoon unsalted butter

¼ teaspoon celery seed

1 teaspoon sea salt

½ teaspoon freshly ground black pepper

Easy-Peel Beets

It is easy to remove the peels from beets. Simply place them in the middle of a large paper towel and rub them until the skin slides off. Gloves are optional but recommended because beets tend to stain everything they come in contact with.

1. Preheat oven to 375°F.

2. Arrange beets in a single layer on a baking sheet. Roast 30 minutes or until fork-tender.

3. Meanwhile, bring a pot of water to a boil. Add celeriac and boil until fork-tender, about 8–20 minutes.

4. Drain and place in a large bowl. Add roasted beets and remaining ingredients. Mash until smooth.

PER SERVING: Calories: 97 | Fat: 2g | Protein: 4g | Sodium: 550mg | Fiber: 3g | Carbohydrates: 16g | Sugar: 4g

Spicy Roasted Spaghetti Squash

Rather than pretend it is pasta, make this dish, which highlights its wonderful squash flavor.

INGREDIENTS | SERVES 4

1 (2-pound) spaghetti squash
2 tablespoons unsalted butter
1 shallot, minced
1 teaspoon salt
½ teaspoon freshly ground black pepper
1 teaspoon ground cayenne
½ teaspoon hot paprika
¼ teaspoon allspice
¼ teaspoon ground cloves

RDA?

RDA stands for recommended daily allowance. The RDA was developed in the 1930s to create standard recommendations of the daily allowance of each type of nutrient. It is meant to reflect the requirements of the majority of the population.

1. Preheat oven to 400°F.

2. Pierce squash with point of a knife multiple times. Place on a baking sheet. Roast 1 hour or until squash is easily pierced with a fork.

3. Halve the squash. Remove seeds and discard. Scoop out the flesh. Shred with a fork. Set aside.

4. Melt butter in a skillet. Add shallot and sauté 2 minutes. Add squash and spices. Sauté an additional 5 minutes. Serve immediately.

PER SERVING: Calories: 71 | Fat: 6g | Protein: 1g | Sodium: 594mg | Fiber: 0g | Carbohydrates: 5g | Sugar: 0g

Pickled Asparagus

This is a type of refrigerator pickling, but this recipe is also safe for hot water bath canning. If you're familiar with hot water bath canning then follow proper safety procedures and process for 10 minutes.

INGREDIENTS | YIELDS 3 PINTS

3½ pounds asparagus, cut into 6" pieces

3 cloves garlic

1 shallot, minced

3 bay leaves

1½ teaspoons black peppercorns

1½ teaspoons dill seeds

1 tablespoon fresh dill

1½ teaspoons yellow mustard seed

2 cups water

2 cups white vinegar

¼ cup pickling salt

1. Evenly divide asparagus, garlic, shallot, bay leaves, peppercorns, dill seeds, dill, and mustard seeds among 3 wide-mouth pint jars.

2. In a saucepan, bring water, vinegar, and salt to a boil, stirring to dissolve salt. Ladle over asparagus. Close jars. Allow jars to come to room temperature and then refrigerate.

3. Wait 1 week before eating. Keep refrigerated at all times.

PER 1-CUP SERVING: Calories: 82 | Fat: 0g | Protein: 6g | Sodium: 4,724mg | Fiber: 6g | Carbohydrates: 14g | Sugar: 5g

Canning

Canning fruits and vegetables is a great way to preserve food at its peak. Pickling is an easy place to start. Even unprocessed pickles keep for months in the refrigerator.

Farro with Rainbow Chard

The chewy texture of the farro contrasts with the more delicate tastes of the chard and fresh herbs.

INGREDIENTS | SERVES 4

4 cups water
1 cup farro
1 shallot, chopped
1 large carrot, diced
1 medium stalk celery, diced
2 cloves garlic, minced
2 tablespoons olive oil
¼ cup chopped Italian parsley
1 bunch rainbow chard, roughly chopped
1½ tablespoons tarragon vinegar

1. Bring 4 cups water and farro to a boil in a medium saucepan over high heat. Reduce heat to low and simmer until tender, stirring occasionally, about 25 minutes. Drain.

2. Meanwhile, sauté shallot, carrot, celery, and garlic in olive oil until the shallots are transparent. Add parsley and chard and sauté until they start to wilt, about 2–3 minutes. Remove from heat. Stir in the farro.

3. Drizzle with vinegar. Serve hot or at room temperature.

PER SERVING: Calories: 259 | Fat: 7g | Protein: 7g | Sodium: 61mg | Fiber: 3g | Carbohydrates: 41g | Sugar: 1g

Viva Farro!

Farro is an ancient grain that is said to be the "mother" of all wheat. It has a nutty flavor and has been popular in Italy since the time when it sustained the Roman legions. Now it is commonly used as an alternative to pasta or rice.

Sage-Parmesan Polenta

Try this creamy polenta at your next meal in place of potatoes, rice, or noodles.

INGREDIENTS | SERVES 4

1 cup polenta

2 cups water or chicken stock

2 cups 2% milk

1 tablespoon unsalted butter

3 ounces grated Parmesan cheese

1 tablespoon minced fresh sage

¼ teaspoon salt

¼ teaspoon freshly ground black pepper

1. Place polenta, water, milk, and butter in a saucepan. Cook on medium heat, whisking occasionally, until thick, about 5–10 minutes.

2. Stir in remaining ingredients. Serve hot.

PER SERVING: Calories: 190 | Fat: 13g | Protein: 12g | Sodium: 374mg | Fiber: 0g | Carbohydrates: 6g | Sugar: 7g

The Creamy Cornmeal

Polenta is a boiled cornmeal dish. It has a thick, creamy texture. Once considered a peasant food, this whole grain has taken on gourmet tendencies. While it was once served plain, it is now common to see it dressed with sauces or enriched with cheese.

Zucchini Boats

Zucchini is a versatile vegetable that takes on whatever flavors it's combined with. This beautiful presentation of zucchini uses all-natural ingredients to create a delicious dish with vibrant colors and flavors for a tasty side or snack.

INGREDIENTS | SERVES 4

4 large zucchini

1 large red bell pepper, seeded and minced

1 medium red onion, peeled and minced

1 cup mushrooms, minced

1 teaspoon garlic powder

1 teaspoon all-natural sea salt

1 teaspoon freshly ground black pepper

1 cup crumbled goat cheese

1. Preheat oven to 400°F and prepare a small oven grate with olive oil spray.

2. Cut zucchini in half lengthwise, and clean seeds out of the center to make a large opening for vegetables.

3. Prepare a large skillet with olive oil spray over medium heat.

4. Sauté pepper, onion, and mushrooms with garlic powder, salt, and pepper until vegetables are slightly softened.

5. Pack sautéed vegetables into the centers of each zucchini, and top with goat cheese.

6. Bake directly on the oven grate 20 minutes, or until zucchini is tender and cheese is melted.

PER SERVING: Calories: 311 | Fat: 21g | Protein: 21g | Sodium: 803mg | Fiber: 4g | Carbohydrates: 13g | Sugar: 9g

Ultimate Spinach and Mushroom Risotto

This delicious risotto is beautiful and amazingly tasty. Sticky long-grain rice makes for a delightfully light yet hearty background to the fresh vegetables.

INGREDIENTS | SERVES 4

1 tablespoon olive oil

1 medium yellow onion, peeled and minced

2 tablespoons minced garlic

1⅓ cups uncooked long-grain brown rice

3¾ cups filtered water

6 cups baby portobello mushrooms, quartered

1 teaspoon all-natural sea salt

1 teaspoon freshly ground black pepper

2 teaspoons Italian seasoning

2 cups baby spinach, chopped

1. Drizzle olive oil in a saucepan over medium heat, and sauté minced onion and garlic until softened, about 5 minutes.

2. Add rice to saucepan and turn to coat in oil, garlic, and onions. Stir over heat 2 minutes.

3. Add water, mushrooms, and seasonings to saucepan, and stir to combine.

4. Bring to a boil, reduce heat to low, and simmer uncovered 20 minutes, stirring frequently.

5. Risotto is done when rice has absorbed all of the liquid, and is sticky but cooked through. Fold in chopped spinach, and stir over heat until the spinach is wilted and combined throughout, about 1–2 minutes.

PER SERVING: Calories: 310 | Fat: 6g | Protein: 9g | Sodium: 618mg | Fiber: 5g | Carbohydrates: 58g | Sugar: 5g

Quinoa with Mixed Vegetables

*As a unique side dish, or a new and exciting entrée, this quinoa recipe
is a quick and easy solution to any dinnertime dilemma.*

INGREDIENTS | SERVES 4

1 cup dry organic quinoa

2 cups filtered water

½ tablespoon garlic powder, divided

½ tablespoon onion powder, divided

½ medium red onion, peeled and chopped

1 cup broccoli florets

1 tablespoon extra-virgin olive oil

1 cup portobello mushrooms

1 teaspoon all-natural sea salt

1. Rinse quinoa thoroughly, and combine with water in a medium saucepan over medium heat and bring to a boil. Reduce heat to low, add half of garlic powder and onion powder, and simmer 15 minutes.

2. In a large sauté pan over medium heat, sauté onion and broccoli in olive oil 7–10 minutes or until slightly softened.

3. Add mushrooms and remaining half of garlic and onion powders to sauté pan and continue cooking until all vegetables are soft.

4. Remove quinoa from heat and transfer to a separate dish. Add sautéed vegetables, and sprinkle with salt to taste.

PER SERVING: Calories: 205 | Fat: 4g | Protein: 8g | Sodium: 602mg | Fiber: 4g | Carbohydrates: 31g | Sugar: 2g

Broccoli-Cauliflower Bake

Fibrous vegetables are an important part of any diet, but most people don't eat enough. This recipe is packed with two favorites—broccoli and cauliflower—and combines them with delicious goat cheese for a flavorful dish brimming with taste and nutrition.

INGREDIENTS | SERVES 4

1 pound broccoli florets

1 pound cauliflower florets

2 tablespoons olive oil

1 cup crumbled goat cheese

What Makes Goat Cheese Superior?

If you're wondering why goat cheese is "clean" but pasteurized processed cheese isn't, it is because of the drastically different makeup of the cheeses. Goat's milk is far superior to that of a cow because there is no need to homogenize goat milk. Goat's milk is naturally homogenized, while cow's milk must be homogenized in the manufacturing process. Without mechanical homogenization, valuable nutrition remains intact and the resulting product has shown to be far less irritating to the human digestive system and less allergenic. In fact, even some lactose-intolerant people are able to consume it without problems.

1. Preheat oven to 375°F and prepare a 13" × 9" casserole dish with olive oil spray.

2. In a large mixing bowl, combine broccoli and cauliflower with olive oil and goat cheese. Mix to coat.

3. Pour mixture into casserole dish, and bake 30–45 minutes, or until vegetables are tender and cheese is melted.

PER SERVING: Calories: 379 | Fat: 28g | Protein: 23g | Sodium: 265mg | Fiber: 5g | Carbohydrates: 14g | Sugar: 5g

Stuffed Mushrooms

These delicious mushrooms can be the perfect appetizer or side dish. Pairing perfectly with fish, meat, vegetables, or pasta, this is a versatile recipe that is quick, easy, and heavenly.

INGREDIENTS | SERVES 6

12 large white mushrooms
½ small zucchini
½ medium red bell pepper
1 teaspoon garlic powder
1 tablespoon filtered water
¼ cup crumbled goat cheese

1. Preheat oven to 375°F. Clean mushrooms with a dry paper towel; remove and reserve stems.

2. Mince zucchini, red pepper, and mushroom stems.

3. Prepare a skillet with olive oil spray over medium heat, and add zucchini and red pepper. Sauté 2–3 minutes; add mushroom stems and garlic powder and continue to sauté until all vegetables are tender.

4. Add water to skillet as needed to prevent sticking and promote steaming.

5. Remove sautéed vegetables from heat and stuff mushroom caps full with mixture. Top with crumbled goat cheese.

6. Place on a nonstick foil-lined baking sheet and bake 20 minutes. Serve hot.

PER SERVING: Calories: 57 | Fat: 4g | Protein: 4g | Sodium: 36mg | Fiber: 1g | Carbohydrates: 3g | Sugar: 2g

Summer Squash Casserole

Packed with vitamin A, this dish is a feast for your eyes and is a perfect side for a low-carbohydrate day.

INGREDIENTS | SERVES 8

1 large zucchini

1 large yellow squash

1 butternut squash

2 tablespoons extra-virgin olive oil

2 tablespoons Italian seasoning

1 tablespoon paprika

2 teaspoons all-natural sea salt

2 cups cooked brown rice

½ cup crumbled goat cheese, or vegan soft cheese

Versatile Deliciousness

If you're looking for a wonderful fresh vegetable that can be made creamy, crunchy, sweet, or salty, look no further than summer squash. Blended with fresh ingredients or light and savory seasonings, you can create incredibly delicious dishes. Whether you'd like a sautéed dish, a hearty casserole, or a creamy soup, summer squash is an easy, inexpensive ingredient that makes for a delicious and nutritious meal any day or night of the week.

1. Cut squashes into bite-sized pieces (strips or rounds) of comparable size.

2. Preheat oven to 400°F and prepare a 13" × 9" baking dish with olive oil spray.

3. In a large mixing bowl, combine squashes, olive oil, and seasonings, and mix well.

4. Fold in rice and goat cheese, place into prepared dish, and bake 35–45 minutes or until cooked through and bubbly.

PER SERVING: Calories: 154 | Fat: 9g | Protein: 6g | Sodium: 640mg | Fiber: 2g | Carbohydrates: 13g | Sugar: 1g

CHAPTER 16

Snacks

No-Bake Apple Crisp
208

Banana Protein Pudding
209

Mocha Protein Bars
209

Triple Berry Parfait
210

Cinnamon Apple Snack Bars
211

Nutty Cottage Cheese
211

Cinnamon Protein Apple Slices
212

Hard-Boiled Eggs
212

Herb Mashed Eggs
213

Protein Guacamole
213

Southwestern Eggs
214

Chocolate-Covered Berry Delight
214

Protein Sludge
215

Garlic Kale Chips
216

No-Bake Apple Crisp

If you enjoy the taste of apple crisp, but not the sugar, fat, and baking process, this simple and fast snack is perfect for you.

INGREDIENTS | SERVES 1

¾ cup nonfat plain Greek yogurt

2 tablespoons unsweetened applesauce

1 medium apple, sliced or diced, peeled if desired

Pinch stevia, or other artificial sweetener

Pinch cinnamon

Pinch nutmeg

Hunger-Fighting Effects of Apples

In addition to being delicious and full of nutrients, apples also contain pectin, a type of fiber that can help you feel full and reduce hunger. If you find yourself feeling hungry between meals and want a healthy snack, reach for an apple.

Mix all ingredients together in a small bowl and enjoy.

PER SERVING: Calories: 220 | Fat: 7g | Protein: 7g | Sodium: 86mg | Fiber: 4g | Carbohydrates: 36g | Sugar: 28g

Banana Protein Pudding

This dish tastes like a luscious dessert and has high protein and electrolytes from the banana to keep you full and energized. Feel free to substitute in any fruit you wish in place of the banana.

INGREDIENTS | SERVES 1

¾ cup nonfat plain Greek yogurt

1 teaspoon fat-free sour cream

½ scoop vanilla protein powder

1 medium banana, sliced

Pinch stevia

Drop vanilla extract

Mix all ingredients together in a small bowl, chill, and enjoy!

PER SERVING: Calories: 264 | Fat: 7g | Protein: 18g | Sodium: 185mg | Fiber: 3g | Carbohydrates: 36g | Sugar: 23g

Mocha Protein Bars

These bars are similar to the Cinnamon Apple Snack Bars in this chapter, except with a chocolate and coffee kick this time.

INGREDIENTS | SERVES 4

¾ cup rolled oats

¼ cup oat bran

6 large egg whites

1 scoop chocolate protein powder

¼ teaspoon baking powder

1 teaspoon cocoa powder

1 tablespoon instant coffee

1 (0.1-ounce) packet stevia

2 medium apples, peeled and diced

1. Preheat oven to 350°F.

2. In a blender, combine all ingredients except apples. Blend until mixture gets thick. Pour mixture into a large bowl.

3. Add apples to mixture and stir to combine.

4. Pour mixture into 9" × 9" baking dish, and bake 30 minutes. Cut into 4 equal bars.

PER SERVING: Calories: 136 | Fat: 2g | Protein: 9g | Sodium: 114mg | Fiber: 4g | Carbohydrates: 25g | Sugar: 9g

Triple Berry Parfait

This recipe has virtually no fat and is incredibly filling thanks to the high protein content.

INGREDIENTS | SERVES 1

¾ cup low-fat plain Greek yogurt

½ scoop vanilla protein powder

⅓ cup blueberries

⅓ cup blackberries

⅓ cup raspberries

Pinch stevia

Drop vanilla extract

Berries: Micronutrient Powerhouses

It's important to hit your macronutrients, of course, but don't ignore those micronutrients. Berries are packed with a variety of antioxidants and micronutrients, so eat a variety of berries as often as you can.

Layer all ingredients together in a small bowl or glass, and serve.

PER SERVING: Calories: 231 | Fat: 4g | Protein: 21g | Sodium: 225mg | Fiber: 6g | Carbohydrates: 30g | Sugar: 22g

Cinnamon Apple Snack Bars

Never buy protein bars again with this recipe. The prep time is well worth the convenience of the finished product.

INGREDIENTS | SERVES 4

¾ cup rolled oats

¼ cup oat bran

6 large egg whites

1 scoop vanilla protein powder (or cinnamon swirl protein)

2 tablespoons unsweetened applesauce

¼ teaspoon baking powder

Pinch stevia

Pinch cinnamon

Drop vanilla extract

2 medium apples, peeled and diced

1. Preheat oven to 350°F.

2. In a blender, combine all ingredients except apples. Blend until mixture gets thick. Pour mixture into a large bowl.

3. Add apples to mixture and stir to combine.

4. Pour mixture into 13" × 9" baking dish and bake 30 minutes. Cut into 4 equal bars.

PER SERVING: Calories: 165 | Fat: 2g | Protein: 15g | Sodium: 124mg | Fiber: 4g | Carbohydrates: 26g | Sugar: 10g

Nutty Cottage Cheese

This recipe contains slow-digesting protein and healthy fats—perfect to keep you full between meals or before bed. Eat with a spoon or dip celery into this mixture.

INGREDIENTS | SERVES 1

½ cup low-fat cottage cheese

1 teaspoon almond butter

1 tablespoon slivered almonds

Pinch stevia

Pinch cinnamon

Mix all ingredients in a small bowl and serve.

PER SERVING: Calories: 162 | Fat: 8g | Protein: 16g | Sodium: 397mg | Fiber: 1g | Carbohydrates: 6g | Sugar: 5g

Cinnamon Protein Apple Slices

These apple slices are quick to make and taste just like apple pie.

INGREDIENTS | SERVES 1

½ scoop vanilla protein powder
1 packet stevia, or other sweetener
¼ teaspoon cinnamon
1 medium apple, peeled and sliced

1. Combine protein powder, stevia, and cinnamon in a sandwich bag or small bowl.

2. Add apple slices, toss until coated, and serve.

PER SERVING: Calories: 129 | Fat: 0g | Protein: 13g | Sodium: 20mg | Fiber: 2g | Carbohydrates: 21g | Sugar: 17g

Hard-Boiled Eggs

Having hard-boiled eggs on hand is an excellent, and very easy, way to get a quick protein fix. They can also be used in other recipes once prepared.

INGREDIENTS | SERVES 6

12 large eggs

1. Place eggs in a single layer in a large saucepan or pot.

2. Cover with just enough cold water to cover eggs by 1".

3. Heat pot over high heat until water starts to boil.

4. Remove pot from burner, cover, and allow eggs to sit 9–12 minutes.

5. Drain immediately, and run eggs under cold water, or chill in ice water, until completely cool.

PER SERVING: Calories: 143 | Fat: 10g | Protein: 13g | Sodium: 140mg | Fiber: 0g | Carbohydrates: 1g | Sugar: 1g

Herb Mashed Eggs

If you have hard-boiled eggs on hand and don't enjoy them plain, here is a quick and easy way to mix it up. You can put this on bread or crackers or eat as is.

INGREDIENTS | SERVES 1

1 whole hard-boiled egg
3 hard-boiled eggs, whites only
1 tablespoon plain nonfat Greek yogurt
Pinch oregano
Pinch parsley
Pinch basil
1 teaspoon olive oil

Add all ingredients to a medium bowl, mash with a fork, and continue to mix until creamy.

PER SERVING: Calories: 115 | Fat: 10g | Protein: 6g | Sodium: 78mg | Fiber: 0g | Carbohydrates: 1g | Sugar: 1g

Protein Guacamole

Guacamole is great as it is, and this variation just adds a little more protein to help you reach your protein goals.

INGREDIENTS | SERVES 1

½ cup low-fat cottage cheese
¼ medium avocado
1 teaspoon salsa
1 teaspoon lemon juice
Pinch garlic powder
Pinch onion powder
Pinch ground cayenne pepper

Combine all ingredients in a medium bowl and mix until smooth.

PER SERVING: Calories: 182 | Fat: 8g | Protein: 15g | Sodium: 413mg | Fiber: 4g | Carbohydrates: 13g | Sugar: 5g

Southwestern Eggs

This quick hard-boiled egg recipe would go great with the Protein Guacamole (see recipe in this chapter) for a complete Southwestern meal.

INGREDIENTS | SERVES 1

1 whole hard-boiled egg
3 hard-boiled eggs, whites only
1 tablespoon plain nonfat Greek yogurt
Pinch chili powder
Pinch garlic powder
Pinch onion powder
1 teaspoon apple cider vinegar

Add all ingredients to a medium bowl, mash with a fork, and continue to mix until creamy.

PER SERVING: Calories: 154 | Fat: 6g | Protein: 19g | Sodium: 270mg | Fiber: 1g | Carbohydrates: 7g | Sugar: 2g

Chocolate-Covered Berry Delight

This takes less than a minute to throw together and tastes absolutely delicious. Not to mention it's extremely high in protein, which will keep you feeling full.

INGREDIENTS | SERVES 1

1 (5.3-ounce) single-serve container mixed berry Greek yogurt
½ scoop chocolate protein powder
¼ cup low-fat whipped cream

1. Mix yogurt and protein powder together in a medium bowl, adding a splash of water if it gets too thick.

2. Top with whipped cream and enjoy. You can also freeze it for a few minutes before serving to chill it.

PER SERVING: Calories: 282 | Fat: 5g | Protein: 22g | Sodium: 160mg | Fiber: 0g | Carbohydrates: 44g | Sugar: 42g

Protein Sludge

Much better than it sounds, this is a very easy and tasty way to consume protein powder if you don't enjoy the taste or texture of mixed protein shakes.

INGREDIENTS | SERVES 1

2 scoops whey protein powder, any flavor

Water, as needed

¼ cup frozen mixed berries, thawed

The Endless Options of Protein Sludge

It can be very hard to hit your protein goals, which is where protein powder can greatly help. If you don't enjoy drinking shakes, sludge is your easiest option, and the variations are endless. Once you have the base sludge of protein and water, you can add anything—berries, oats, nuts, peanut butter, whipped cream, rice cakes, or anything else you can think of.

1. Place protein powder in a bowl.

2. Add a splash of water, stir well, and repeat until protein is the consistency of a thick pudding.

3. Add mixed berries and any other toppings you want, and enjoy.

PER SERVING: Calories: 231 | Fat: 1g | Protein: 50g | Sodium: 80mg | Fiber: 1g | Carbohydrates: 7g | Sugar: 6g

Garlic Kale Chips

Kale is one of the most nutritious vegetables you can eat, perhaps even more nutritious than spinach. It has incredible health benefits and this recipe turns it into a delicious snack.

INGREDIENTS | SERVES 1

2 cups whole raw kale leaves
1 tablespoon olive oil
¼ teaspoon garlic salt
1 tablespoon grated Parmesan cheese

1. Preheat oven to 400°F.

2. Wash kale and tear into smaller pieces.

3. Once kale is thoroughly dry, mix with olive oil in a large bowl, making sure all pieces are coated.

4. Spread out evenly on baking sheet covered with aluminum foil.

5. Sprinkle with garlic salt and cheese.

6. Bake 8–12 minutes, or until it reaches your desired crispness.

PER SERVING: Calories: 213 | Fat: 16g | Protein: 7g | Sodium: 742mg | Fiber: 3g | Carbohydrates: 14g | Sugar: 0g

CHAPTER 17

Holidays

Spice-Rubbed Roasted Turkey
Breast
218

Pressure Cooker Beef
Bourguignon
219

Pork Loin with Baked Apples
220

Whole-Grain Rotini with Pork,
Pumpkin, and Sage
221

Shrimp Creole
222

Shepherd's Pie
223

Roasted Radishes and Brussels
Sprouts
224

Vegetable Baked Ziti
225

Oyster Portobello Un-Stuffing
226

Garlic Rosemary Mashed
Potatoes
227

Whipped Sweet Potatoes
228

Mushroom Barley Pilaf with
Fresh Green Beans
229

Roasted Root Vegetables with
Orange and Thyme
230

Buttermilk Biscuits
231

Rosemary Wild Rice Pilaf
232

Shrimp Shiitake Pot Stickers
233

Goat Cheese–Stuffed Dates
234

Sweet and Spicy Almonds
235

Apple, Pear, and Cranberry
Crisp with Fresh Ginger
236

Chocolate Pomegranate
Brownies
237

Pound Cake Minis
238

Spice-Rubbed Roasted Turkey Breast

Turkey breast gets a bad reputation for being bland. Yet it's protein-packed and can be made as flavorful as you want. This recipe combines an abundance of spices that will kick up the flavors at your holiday table.

INGREDIENTS | SERVES 8

1 (5-pound) turkey breast
2 teaspoons garlic powder
2 teaspoons onion powder
1 teaspoon cayenne
1 teaspoon all-natural sea salt
1 teaspoon freshly ground black pepper
1 tablespoon olive oil
1 large lemon, sliced

1. Preheat oven to 325°F, and prepare a roasting pan with olive oil spray. Set turkey breast in roasting pan (if previously frozen, make sure it is thawed).

2. Combine all spices in a small mixing bowl, and mix well.

3. Coat turkey breast with olive oil, and sprinkle spice mixture over turkey breast. Top with lemon slices.

4. Cook turkey breast 1½–2½ hours, or until internal temperature reads 165–170°F. Slice and serve hot.

PER SERVING: Calories: 331 | Fat: 4g | Protein: 69g | Sodium: 433mg | Fiber: 1g | Carbohydrates: 2g | Sugar: 0g

Pressure Cooker Beef Bourguignon

A simple lower-sodium take on the traditional French dish. The pressure cooker cuts cooking time by two-thirds, leaving this ready in just 30 minutes! The heavenly smell of simmering beef and onions will have you (and your lucky guests) salivating.

INGREDIENTS | SERVES 6

2 tablespoons unsalted butter

3 large onions, peeled and sliced

2 pounds lean beef stew meat, cubed

2 cups water

1½ cups red wine

2 teaspoons sodium-free beef bouillon granules

½ teaspoon dried marjoram

½ teaspoon dried thyme

½ teaspoon freshly ground black pepper

1 pound white mushrooms, thickly sliced

Pressure Cookers

Pressure cookers are amazing tools. Not only do they speed cooking time and allow you to make meals fast, they retain more nutrients and are one of the most environmentally friendly means of cooking. Opt for a stainless steel appliance, which won't pit from acids in lemon juice, vinegar, and the like.

1. Melt butter in pressure cooker over medium-high heat. Add onions and cook, stirring, 5 minutes.

2. Move onions to side of pan, add cubed beef, and brown on all sides, about 5 minutes.

3. Add remaining ingredients and stir to combine. Secure the lid on the pressure cooker and set to high. Raise the heat to high and bring contents to a boil. Once you hear sizzling, reduce heat to medium and cook 20 minutes.

4. Remove from heat. Allow pressure cooker to depressurize naturally, or place under cold running water for about 5 minutes. Serve immediately.

PER SERVING: Calories: 401 | Fat: 19g | Protein: 34g | Sodium: 115mg | Fiber: 2g | Carbohydrates: 12g | Sugar: 5g

Pork Loin with Baked Apples

Rather than dipping your pork in applesauce, why not build apples into the meal itself? Aromatic, tasty, and satisfying, this delicious combination of salty pork and sweet baked apples will surely become one of your family's favorites.

INGREDIENTS | SERVES 4

¼ cup unsweetened applesauce

2 tablespoons filtered water

3 medium gala apples, cored, peeled, and cut into slices

1 teaspoon cinnamon

1 pound pork tenderloin

1 teaspoon all-natural sea salt

1 tablespoon agave nectar

1. Preheat oven to 400°F and spray a 13" × 9" pan with olive oil spray.

2. Mix applesauce, water, and apples in a mixing bowl with cinnamon.

3. Layer apples evenly in the pan, and cook 20 minutes, or until slightly softened.

4. Place pork tenderloin in the middle of the pan and surround with apples.

5. Sprinkle tenderloin with sea salt, and drizzle agave nectar over the pork and the apples.

6. Return pan to oven for another 30 minutes, or until the internal temperature reads 165°F.

PER SERVING: Calories: 204 | Fat: 3g | Protein: 24g | Sodium: 650mg | Fiber: 2g | Carbohydrates: 22g | Sugar: 18g

Whole-Grain Rotini with Pork, Pumpkin, and Sage

A deliciously filling main dish. The pumpkin adds color, nutrients, and subtle flavor. Rotini, corkscrew-shaped pasta with a lot of surface area, allows the sauce to really cling. Feel free to substitute a different variety of pasta if you prefer.

INGREDIENTS | SERVES 6

1 (13-ounce) package whole-grain rotini

1 pound lean ground pork

1 medium red onion, peeled and diced

3 cloves garlic, minced

1 medium bell pepper, diced

1 cup pumpkin purée

2 teaspoons ground sage

1 teaspoon ground rosemary

½–1 teaspoon freshly ground black pepper

1. Cook pasta according to package directions. Drain and set aside.

2. Heat sauté pan over medium heat. Add ground pork, onion, and garlic and sauté 2 minutes.

3. Add bell pepper and sauté 5 minutes.

4. Remove from heat. Add pasta to pan along with remaining ingredients. Stir well to combine. Serve immediately.

PER SERVING: Calories: 331 | Fat: 7g | Protein: 23g | Sodium: 48mg | Fiber: 8g | Carbohydrates: 45g | Sugar: 3g

Shrimp Creole

This spicy and beautiful shrimp dish features amazing flavors, perfect for special occasions. Serve over cooked brown or white rice.

INGREDIENTS | SERVES 6

2 teaspoons canola oil

1 medium onion, peeled and thinly sliced

1 medium bell pepper, thinly sliced

2 medium stalks celery, thinly sliced

3 cloves garlic, minced

2 (15-ounce) cans no-salt-added diced tomatoes

1 (8-ounce) can no-salt-added tomato sauce

⅓ cup white wine

½ teaspoon apple cider vinegar

2 bay leaves

2 teaspoons salt-free chili seasoning

1 teaspoon ground sweet paprika

½ teaspoon freshly ground black pepper

⅛ teaspoon ground cayenne pepper

1 pound peeled shrimp, tails removed

1. Heat oil in sauté pan over medium heat. Add onion, bell pepper, celery, and garlic and cook, stirring, 5 minutes.

2. Add remaining ingredients except shrimp and stir well to combine. Simmer 10 minutes, stirring frequently. Cover and reduce heat to medium-low if sauce begins to splatter.

3. Stir in the shrimp and simmer 5 minutes.

4. Remove from heat and remove bay leaves from pan. Serve immediately.

PER SERVING: Calories: 152 | Fat: 3g | Protein: 17g | Sodium: 136mg | Fiber: 2g | Carbohydrates: 11g | Sugar: 6g

The Skinny on Shrimp

Shrimp come in a variety of sizes, from miniscule to extra colossal, and are typically sold by weight and size; for instance, a pound of large shrimp contains roughly 30–35 pieces. Most shrimp consumed in the United States have been processed to some degree and may have added salt. Read package labels carefully and buy fresh, unprocessed shrimp whenever possible.

Shepherd's Pie

This classic family favorite was begging for a clean makeover. This recipe's unique blend of spices and clean ingredients give you all the comforting flavor you love without the fat and calories you don't. Enjoy it tonight, then freeze the leftovers!

INGREDIENTS | SERVES 16

1 pound Idaho potatoes, peeled, washed, and cubed

1 pound cauliflower florets

4 teaspoons garlic powder, divided

4 teaspoons onion powder, divided

2 teaspoons all-natural sea salt, divided

2 teaspoons freshly ground black pepper, divided

2 cups unsweetened almond milk

2 pounds browned ground turkey breast

1 medium onion, peeled and minced

4 cups frozen peas

Flavorful Turkey Breast

Turkey has long been considered the healthier alternative to other meats because of its lower saturated fat content. Spices, not fat, make for tasty turkey meat. So forget about using the "juices" of beef's fat to marinate and tenderize—instead, use turkey and baste and marinate with spices instead. With turkey, you don't sacrifice flavor for health.

1. In large pot over medium heat, bring potato cubes to a boil, reduce heat to low, and simmer 10 minutes.

2. Add cauliflower to the pot and simmer for an additional 10 minutes, or until the cauliflower is fork-tender.

3. Remove pot from the heat, drain, and move the potatoes and cauliflower to a large serving bowl. Season with 2 teaspoons garlic powder, 1 teaspoon onion powder, 1 teaspoon salt, and 1 teaspoon pepper.

4. Mash or beat the potatoes and cauliflower, adding almond milk ¼ cup at a time until desired texture is achieved.

5. Preheat oven to 350°F and spray a 13" × 9" dish with olive oil spray.

6. In a mixing bowl, combine browned ground turkey breast, half of the minced onion, 2 teaspoons garlic powder, 2 teaspoons onion powder, 1 teaspoon salt, and 1 teaspoon pepper, and blend well.

7. Layer the meat on the bottom of the pan, cover with the peas, and sprinkle with the remaining minced onion.

8. Spoon mashed potatoes and cauliflower over the peas, spreading evenly.

9. Bake 30 minutes, or until mashed cauliflower begins to turn golden.

PER SERVING: Calories: 149 | Fat: 2g | Protein: 18g | Sodium: 462mg | Fiber: 2g | Carbohydrates: 17g | Sugar: 3g

Roasted Radishes and Brussels Sprouts

The roasting process mellows the flavor of both vegetables, leaving them ultra-tender and caramelized. The pepper gains strength in the oven; use the lesser amount if you can't tolerate spice.

INGREDIENTS | SERVES 4

½ pound radishes

1 pound Brussels sprouts, halved

1 tablespoon freshly squeezed lemon juice

1½ teaspoons olive oil

¼–½ teaspoon freshly ground black pepper

Radish Facts

Radishes, like carrots, are root vegetables. Radishes and radish greens, as their edible leaves are known, have a pungent, peppery taste. This, along with their often vibrant colors, makes them a great choice for accenting salads. Roasting, braising, sautéing, or steaming radishes mellows their flavor significantly. Radishes are high in vitamin C and fiber and low in calories and sodium.

1. Preheat oven to 425°F. Spray a baking sheet lightly with oil and set aside.

2. Wash radishes and pat dry. Halve or quarter depending upon size and place into a mixing bowl.

3. Add halved Brussels sprouts, lemon juice, oil, and pepper and toss well to coat.

4. Arrange in a single layer on baking sheet. Place on middle rack in oven and bake 25–30 minutes.

5. Remove from oven and serve immediately.

PER SERVING: Calories: 64 | Fat: 2g | Protein: 3g | Sodium: 45mg | Fiber: 3g | Carbohydrates: 10g | Sugar: 3g

Vegetable Baked Ziti

Delicious comfort food at its best, this version of baked ziti is packed with fresh vegetables. Water-packed mozzarella is often sold in the specialty cheese section of supermarkets. It's softer and much lower in sodium than its dry counterparts. If you can't find it, substitute shredded Swiss cheese instead.

INGREDIENTS | SERVES 6

1 pound dry whole-grain ziti

1 tablespoon olive oil

1 medium onion, peeled and diced

4 cloves garlic, minced

1 medium bell pepper, diced

1 medium yellow squash, diced

1 medium zucchini, diced

1 (15-ounce) can no-salt-added diced tomatoes

2 (8-ounce) cans no-salt-added tomato sauce

2 tablespoons tomato paste

1 teaspoon brown sugar

1 teaspoon dried basil

½ teaspoon dried marjoram

½ teaspoon dried oregano

½ teaspoon freshly ground black pepper

¼ teaspoon dried savory

¼ teaspoon dried thyme

4 ounces fresh water-packed mozzarella cheese, shredded

2 tablespoons grated Parmesan cheese

1. Preheat oven to 400°F. Get out a 13" × 9" baking pan and set aside.

2. Cook ziti according to package directions. Drain and set aside.

3. Heat oil in a sauté pan over medium heat. Add onion and garlic and sauté 2 minutes.

4. Add bell pepper, squash, zucchini, tomatoes with juice, tomato sauce, tomato paste, brown sugar, and seasonings and cook, stirring, 10 minutes. Remove from heat.

5. Pour sauce into the pot of pasta. Add cheeses and stir to combine. Pour mixture into the baking dish. Cover tightly with aluminum foil. Place pan on middle rack in oven and bake 20 minutes.

6. Remove from oven and let rest 5 minutes before serving.

PER SERVING: Calories: 384 | Fat: 8g | Protein: 17g | Sodium: 180mg | Fiber: 11g | Carbohydrates: 65g | Sugar: 10g

Oyster Portobello Un-Stuffing

A twist on traditional stuffing, this stuffing is made into balls and cooks in the pan next to your turkey, not inside it.

INGREDIENTS | SERVES 10

3 tablespoons unsalted butter

1 pound celery, chopped

1 pound onions, chopped

4 portobello mushroom caps, diced

1 bunch parsley, minced

25 slices torn sandwich bread

2 large eggs, beaten

1 teaspoon freshly ground black pepper

1 teaspoon sea salt

1 teaspoon celery seed

1 teaspoon paprika

16 ounces shucked oysters, liquid reserved

½ cup chicken stock

Turkey or chicken in the process of being roasted

1. Melt the butter in large skillet. Add celery, onions, and mushrooms and cook over very low heat until onions are translucent but not browned, about 30–45 minutes. Allow to cool slightly. Sprinkle with parsley.

2. Scrape the mixture into a large bowl. Add remaining ingredients. Using your hands, mix ingredients together until all ingredients are evenly distributed.

3. Form mixture into 3" balls that hold their shape. If the balls do not hold their shape, add the reserved oyster liquor until they can hold their shape.

4. Place balls in the bottom of the roasting pan under the rack and around the turkey (or chicken) and return to the oven for the last ½ hour of roasting.

PER SERVING: Calories: 290 | Fat: 10g | Protein: 11g | Sodium: 1,042mg | Fiber: 4g | Carbohydrates: 45g | Sugar: 6g

Garlic Rosemary Mashed Potatoes

Potatoes often fall flat without additional flavors, but these mashed potatoes, made with garlic, rosemary, rice wine vinegar, pepper, and mustard, may be the best you've ever had.

INGREDIENTS | SERVES 6

6 cups cubed red potatoes

6 cloves garlic

2 tablespoons olive oil

¼ cup low-sodium vegetable broth

1 teaspoon unflavored rice wine vinegar

1 teaspoon ground rosemary

½ teaspoon ground white pepper

¼ teaspoon ground dry mustard

Rosemary Facts

Rosemary is a perennial herb with a strong taste and fragrance. It grows in sturdy sprigs with leaves reminiscent of soft pine needles. Rosemary can be used either fresh or dried, and is often ground into a fragrant powder for ease in use. It contains iron and several antioxidants believed to ward against neurological disorders such as Alzheimer's and Parkinson's disease.

1. Place potatoes in a pot and add enough water to cover. Place pot over high heat and bring to a boil. Once boiling, reduce heat to medium-high and simmer 15 minutes.

2. Measure remaining ingredients into a food processor and purée until smooth.

3. Remove pot from heat and drain. Mash potatoes. Add dressing and stir well to combine.

4. Serve immediately.

PER SERVING: Calories: 181 | Fat: 4g | Protein: 3g | Sodium: 13mg | Fiber: 3g | Carbohydrates: 32g | Sugar: 1g

Whipped Sweet Potatoes

Perfect for holiday meals, this light and creamy concoction of sweet potato has hints of orange and vanilla.

INGREDIENTS | SERVES 6

3 medium–large sweet potatoes

3 tablespoons unsalted butter

3 tablespoons brown sugar

1 tablespoon freshly squeezed orange juice

¼ teaspoon pure vanilla extract

Whipped Butternut Squash

Puréed winter squash is a favorite recipe in New England and is super easy to make. Peel a medium butternut squash, seed, then cut into chunks. Place chunks in a microwave-safe bowl, add ¼ cup water, and cover with plastic wrap. Microwave on high for 10 minutes. Transfer contents to a food processor, add a tablespoon of low-sodium chicken or vegetable broth, and purée. Season to taste.

1. Peel sweet potatoes and cut into chunks. Place chunks in a pot and add enough water to cover by 1–2". Place pot over high heat and bring to a boil. Once boiling, lower heat slightly and continue cooking until tender, about 20 minutes.

2. Drain pot. Place ⅓ of the sweet potatoes into a food processor, add 1 tablespoon butter, and purée. Remove to a bowl. Repeat process with remaining sweet potatoes and butter.

3. Add the brown sugar, orange juice, and vanilla to the bowl of whipped sweet potatoes and stir well to combine. Serve immediately.

PER SERVING: Calories: 136 | Fat: 5g | Protein: 1g | Sodium: 23mg | Fiber: 2g | Carbohydrates: 20g | Sugar: 11g

Mushroom Barley Pilaf with Fresh Green Beans

This quick, healthy, and filling side also makes a great vegetarian main course. Quick barley speeds cooking time, getting this to the table in just 20 minutes. Substitute an equal amount of sliced garlic scapes for the garlic and green beans when in season.

INGREDIENTS | SERVES 4

1 cup dry quick barley

2 cups boiling water

1 teaspoon olive oil

1 medium red onion, peeled and diced

4 cloves garlic, minced

8 ounces fresh mushrooms, sliced

1 cup fresh green beans, cut into 1" pieces

¼ teaspoon dried marjoram

¼ teaspoon dried thyme

¼ teaspoon freshly ground black pepper

What Is Barley?

Barley is a type of whole grain, with a chewy texture and slightly nutty taste. Regular pearled barley cooks in about 40 minutes; quick barley is parboiled, allowing it to cook in a quarter of the time. Most of the barley grown in the United States is destined for beverages rather than food. Fermented barley, also known as barley malt, is an important ingredient in beer making. Barley is cholesterol free, low in fat, and high in fiber.

1. Measure barley into a saucepan and stir in boiling water. Place over high heat and bring to a boil. Once boiling, reduce heat to low, cover, and simmer 10 minutes. Drain excess water and set aside.

2. Heat oil in a sauté pan over medium heat. Add onion and garlic and sauté 2 minutes.

3. Add mushrooms and green beans and sauté 5 minutes.

4. Remove from heat. Stir in barley and seasonings. Serve immediately.

PER SERVING: Calories: 183 | Fat: 2g | Protein: 5g | Sodium: 8mg | Fiber: 6g | Carbohydrates: 38g | Sugar: 2g

Roasted Root Vegetables with Orange and Thyme

*A beautiful vegetable medley with a bright color and taste. Cut the
vegetables into equal-sized pieces to ensure even cooking.*

INGREDIENTS | SERVES 6

3 medium carrots

3 medium parsnips

2 medium sweet potatoes

3 tablespoons freshly squeezed
orange juice

1 tablespoon olive oil

1 tablespoon fresh thyme or
1 teaspoon dried

¼ teaspoon freshly ground black pepper

Thyme Time

Thyme is an easy-to-grow perennial herb.
Its strong, distinct flavor makes it a great
choice for many types of roasts, soups, and
stews. When using fresh thyme, gently run
your fingers along its woody stem, removing the leaves. Leaves may be added whole
or chopped. If fresh thyme is not available,
dried thyme is a good alternative.

1. Preheat oven to 450°F. Take out a sided baking sheet and set aside.

2. Peel vegetables and cut into 1" pieces. Place in a mixing bowl, add remaining ingredients, and toss well to coat.

3. Turn mixture out onto baking sheet and arrange vegetables in a single layer.

4. Place baking sheet on middle rack in oven and bake 30 minutes.

5. Remove from oven and serve immediately.

PER SERVING: Calories: 123 | Fat: 2g | Protein: 2g |
Sodium: 43mg | Fiber: 5g | Carbohydrates: 24g | Sugar: 7g

Buttermilk Biscuits

What goes better with a holiday dinner than buttermilk biscuits?

INGREDIENTS | SERVES 10

1½ cups all-purpose flour

1½ teaspoons baking powder

1 teaspoon baking soda

1 teaspoon sugar

½ teaspoon salt

6 tablespoons cold unsalted butter, sliced

½ cup buttermilk

1 large egg

1. Preheat oven to 350°F.

2. Pulse flour, baking powder, baking soda, sugar, and salt in a food processor. Add butter and pulse until just mixed.

3. In a small bowl, beat together buttermilk and egg. Pour into the food processor and pulse until a dough forms.

4. Place the dough on a floured surface and knead briefly. Roll out into a ½" thickness. Cut with biscuit cutter. Place on a parchment paper–lined baking sheet.

5. Bake 10 minutes or until golden brown.

PER SERVING: Calories: 239 | Fat: 13g | Protein: 5g | Sodium: 563mg | Fiber: 1g | Carbohydrates: 26g | Sugar: 2g

Rosemary Wild Rice Pilaf

Wild rice provides a nutty flavor and chewy texture to this pilaf.

INGREDIENTS | SERVES 10

3½ cups water

1 cup brown rice

½ cup wild rice

1 medium onion, peeled and chopped

2 medium stalks celery, chopped

2 medium carrots, diced

1 bulb fennel, diced

3 tablespoons chopped rosemary

½ teaspoon salt

½ teaspoon freshly ground black pepper

1. In a medium pot, bring the water to a boil. Add brown rice and wild rice. Cook until tender, about 45 minutes.

2. Meanwhile, spray a skillet with nonstick cooking spray. Sauté onion, celery, carrots, and fennel until softened.

3. Preheat oven to 350°F.

4. Drain the rice and wild rice. Pour into an 8" × 8" baking dish. Stir in the vegetable mixture. Cover and bake 1 hour. Add spices. Fluff with a fork prior to serving.

PER SERVING: Calories: 73 | Fat: 1g | Protein: 2g | Sodium: 148mg | Fiber: 3g | Carbohydrates: 16g | Sugar: 1g

America's Grain

First harvested by Native Americans, wild rice is one of the very few grains native to North America. Despite the name, wild rice is actually a grain harvested from a type of grass, not rice. It grows in shallow lakes and streams. Wild rice is the state grain of Minnesota.

Shrimp Shiitake Pot Stickers

Homemade pot stickers are easier to make than you might think, and unlike their supermarket counterparts, they are full of fresh ingredients and are preservative free.

INGREDIENTS | SERVES 25

1 large whole egg

1 bunch scallions, minced

4 fresh shiitake mushrooms, minced

2 heads baby bok choy, finely chopped

1 pound raw shrimp, deveined and minced

2 tablespoons sesame oil

2 tablespoons soy sauce

2 tablespoons grated fresh ginger

1½ tablespoons grated garlic

1½ tablespoons cornstarch

1 teaspoon finely ground fresh black pepper

50 round dumpling wrappers

5 cups water

Easy Dumpling Dipping Sauce

Wow guests with this homemade sauce. Simply whisk together ¼ cup soy sauce, ¼ cup rice wine vinegar, 1½ teaspoons sesame oil, and ½ teaspoon chili garlic sauce. Garnish with chopped scallions if desired.

1. In a large bowl, combine egg, scallions, mushrooms, bok choy, shrimp, sesame oil, soy sauce, ginger, garlic, cornstarch, and pepper to form a uniform mixture.

2. Place a dumpling wrapper on a plate or clean, dry surface. Place a teaspoon of filling in the center of the dumpling wrapper. Fold the wrapper in half to form a half-moon shape, pinching the wrapper tightly together. Press the "fold" side gently down on the plate so it can stand alone, seam side up. Repeat until all of the filling and wrappers are gone.

3. Heat a small amount of canola oil in a large saucepan over medium heat. Place about 10 pot stickers flat side down and fry until the bottom is browned. Add 1 cup of water; cover immediately. Allow dumplings to steam about 5–10 minutes.

4. Once the dumplings are fully cooked the water will have fully evaporated and the bottoms will be crisp. Repeat for remaining dumplings.

PER SERVING: Calories: 89 | Fat: 2g | Protein: 7g | Sodium: 237mg | Fiber: 1g | Carbohydrates: 12g | Sugar: 1g

Goat Cheese–Stuffed Dates

Gooey dates are the perfect foil for the zesty, savory filling.

INGREDIENTS | SERVES 8

½ pound pitted Medjool dates

4 ounces soft goat cheese, at room temperature

2 tablespoons lemon zest

¼ teaspoon salt

¼ teaspoon ground culinary lavender

Darling Dates

One serving of Medjool dates contains 3 grams of fiber and is a great source of potassium, iron, magnesium, and calcium. Despite their sweetness, their glycemic index is only a 9. They also contain the anti-oxidants zeaxanthin, lutein, and beta carotene.

1. Slice each date lengthwise to make an opening without cutting all the way through. Set aside.

2. In a small bowl, stir together cheese, zest, salt, and lavender. Spoon an equal amount into each date. Serve immediately or refrigerate.

PER SERVING: Calories: 142 | Fat: 5g | Protein: 5g | Sodium: 123mg | Fiber: 2g | Carbohydrates: 21g | Sugar: 18g

Sweet and Spicy Almonds

Tastes like dessert but it is actually an excellent source of good fats and protein.

INGREDIENTS | SERVES 8

1 tablespoon olive oil

2 cups whole almonds

1 tablespoon sugar

1 teaspoon cayenne pepper

1 teaspoon chipotle powder

½ teaspoon chili powder

Awesome Almonds

Almonds are an excellent source of vitamin E, a powerful antioxidant that helps protect the skin from oxygen free radicals. Almonds are also a good source of fiber. 100 grams of almonds also contains 25 percent of the daily recommended dose of calcium.

1. Preheat oven to 250°F. Line two baking sheets with parchment paper.

2. Toss all ingredients together. Make sure the nuts are evenly coated.

3. Arrange in a single layer on one of the baking sheets and bake 25 minutes, or until the almonds look mostly dry, stirring every 5 minutes.

4. Remove from the oven. Pour onto the remaining lined baking sheet to cool.

PER SERVING: Calories: 158 | Fat: 13g | Protein: 5g | Sodium: 1mg | Fiber: 3g | Carbohydrates: 7g | Sugar: 3g

Apple, Pear, and Cranberry Crisp with Fresh Ginger

*Juicy fruit under a sweet whole-grain crust. What's not to love? This fabulous
crisp is a perfect vehicle for fall fruit. Vary the types of apples and pears to subtly
change the flavor, or swap them altogether for a different fruit or fruits.*

INGREDIENTS | SERVES 8

3 medium apples

3 medium pears

1 cup fresh or frozen cranberries

1 tablespoon freshly squeezed
lemon juice

2 tablespoons minced fresh ginger

⅓ cup sugar

1 cup rolled oats

⅓ cup white whole-wheat flour

½ cup light brown sugar

1 teaspoon pure vanilla extract

1 teaspoon ground cinnamon

¼ teaspoon ground allspice

⅛ teaspoon ground cardamom

3 tablespoons unsalted butter

Freezer Alert

Fresh cranberries are often on sale around
the holidays. Buy an extra bag or two and
pop them into the freezer for future use. If
kept frozen, cranberries will last for months
and can be added to many recipes, often
without defrosting.

1. Preheat oven to 400°F. Take out a 2-quart baking pan
   and set aside.

2. Peel and core apples and pears, and slice each into
   16 wedges.

3. Place into a mixing bowl, add cranberries, lemon juice,
   ginger, and sugar and toss well to coat.

4. Turn mixture out into the baking pan and set aside.

5. Place oats, flour, sugar, vanilla, and spices into a
   mixing bowl and stir to combine.

6. Cut butter into the mixture using your (freshly washed)
   hands and process until a wet crumb has formed.
   Sprinkle mixture over fruit.

7. Place on middle rack in oven and bake 30 minutes.
   Remove from oven and place on a wire rack to cool.

PER SERVING: Calories: 263 | Fat: 5g | Protein: 2g |
Sodium: 6mg | Fiber: 6g | Carbohydrates: 55g | Sugar: 36g

Chocolate Pomegranate Brownies

Moist with an undeniably decadent taste, every bite of these brownies is infused with the dark sweetness of pomegranate juice. These make a spectacular treat for special occasions.

INGREDIENTS | SERVES 16

¾ cup unsweetened cocoa powder

¾ cup unbleached all-purpose flour

¾ cup sugar

1 cup pomegranate juice (e.g., POM Wonderful)

2 large whole eggs

½ cup canola oil

1 teaspoon sodium-free baking powder

1. Preheat oven to 350°F. Grease and flour an 8" square pan and set aside.

2. Place ingredients into a mixing bowl and beat 2 minutes.

3. Pour batter into prepared pan. Place pan on middle rack in oven and bake 30 minutes.

4. Remove from oven and place on wire rack to cool. Cool to touch before cutting into squares and serving.

PER SERVING: (Per Brownie) Calories: 144 | Fat: 8g | Protein: 2g | Sodium: 11mg | Fiber: 1g | Carbohydrates: 18g | Sugar: 11g

Pound Cake Minis

Save these rich little cakes for a seriously special occasion. Although healthier than classic pound cake, they're still pretty decadent.

INGREDIENTS | SERVES 18

½ cup unsalted butter

¼ cup nonhydrogenated vegetable shortening

1 cup sugar

2 egg whites

2 teaspoons pure vanilla extract

¼ teaspoon pure almond extract

½ teaspoon sodium-free baking powder

1¼ cups unbleached all-purpose flour

½ cup low-fat milk

1. Preheat oven to 350°F. Line 18 muffin cups with paper liners and set aside.

2. Place butter and shortening into a mixing bowl.

3. Add sugar and beat until fluffy.

4. Beat in egg whites and extracts.

5. Stir in baking powder and gradually add in flour, alternating with milk, and stir until combined.

6. Spoon batter into muffin tins, filling each cup about ⅔ full. Place muffin tins on middle rack in oven and bake 20 minutes.

7. Remove from oven and transfer to a wire rack to cool.

PER SERVING: Calories: 150 | Fat: 8g | Protein: 1g | Sodium: 10mg | Fiber: 0g | Carbohydrates: 18g | Sugar: 11g

CHAPTER 18

Drinks

Cinnamon Chai Latte Smoothie
240

Neapolitan Smoothie
241

Blue Velvet Smoothie
241

Mint Chocolate Chip Smoothie
242

Key Lime Pie Smoothie
242

Orange Cream Delight
243

Peaches and Cream Smoothie
243

Protein Piña Colada
244

Peanut Butter and Jelly Smoothie
244

Tiramisu Smoothie
245

Chocolate Peanut Butter Cup Smoothie
245

Tropical Blend Smoothie
246

Pumpkin Pie Protein Shake
246

Super Greens Shake
247

Cinnamon Chai Latte Smoothie

This smoothie combines the delicious and refreshing taste of chai with protein for a low-calorie, filling drink.

INGREDIENTS | SERVES 1

1 scoop vanilla protein powder

1 cup cold cinnamon chai tea

Pinch stevia

Pinch cinnamon

5 ice cubes

Combine all ingredients in a blender and process until smooth. Serve immediately.

PER SERVING: Calories: 6 | Fat: 0g | Protein: 0g | Sodium: 0mg | Fiber: 1g | Carbohydrates: 2g | Sugar: 0g

A Quick Word on Protein Powder

The drinks in this section contain protein powder. Drinking protein smoothies will keep you full, and make it very easy to hit your daily protein goals, something many struggle with. You can choose any flavor you like, and you'll want to look for a protein with minimal ingredients. Whey protein works best for these recipes.

Neapolitan Smoothie

The classic combination of chocolate, vanilla, and strawberry—what's not to love?

INGREDIENTS | SERVES 1

1 scoop vanilla protein powder

3–4 frozen strawberries

1 teaspoon cocoa powder

Pinch stevia

5 ice cubes

Combine all ingredients in a blender and process until smooth. Serve immediately.

PER SERVING: Calories: 124 | Fat: 1g | Protein: 26g | Sodium: 41mg | Fiber: 1g | Carbohydrates: 6g | Sugar: 3g

Blue Velvet Smoothie

This smoothie is fruity, chocolaty, and loaded with antioxidants to keep you healthy.

INGREDIENTS | SERVES 1

1 scoop chocolate protein powder

½ cup low-fat plain Greek yogurt

½ cup fresh blueberries

1 teaspoon cocoa powder

Pinch stevia

5 ice cubes

Combine all ingredients in a blender and process until smooth. Serve immediately.

PER SERVING: Calories: 228 | Fat: 3g | Protein: 32g | Sodium: 127mg | Fiber: 2g | Carbohydrates: 21g | Sugar: 17g

Mint Chocolate Chip Smoothie

This smoothie is cold and refreshing, perfect for a hot summer day.
It's like having your favorite ice cream in a glass.

INGREDIENTS | SERVES 1

1 scoop chocolate protein powder
1 teaspoon mint extract
½ cup skim milk
1 cup cold water
1 teaspoon cocoa powder
Pinch stevia
5 ice cubes

Combine all ingredients in a blender and process until smooth. Serve immediately.

PER SERVING: Calories: 160 | Fat: 2g | Protein: 29g | Sodium: 101mg | Fiber: 1g | Carbohydrates: 8g | Sugar: 7g

Key Lime Pie Smoothie

A refreshing, tropical smoothie—all the taste of the classic dessert without all the guilt and calories.

INGREDIENTS | SERVES 1

1 scoop vanilla protein powder
½ cup lime juice
½ cup low-fat cottage cheese
1 medium banana
5 ice cubes

Combine all ingredients in a blender and process until smooth. Serve immediately.

PER SERVING: Calories: 317 | Fat: 4g | Protein: 40g | Sodium: 414mg | Fiber: 4g | Carbohydrates: 36g | Sugar: 20g

Orange Cream Delight

With a whole orange, this smoothie contains loads of vitamin C and some natural carbs and sugar. This one is great to enjoy after a run outside or a tough workout.

INGREDIENTS | SERVES 1

1 scoop vanilla protein powder
½ cup plain nonfat Greek yogurt
1 peeled and separated frozen orange
1 cup cold water

Combine all ingredients in a blender and process until smooth. Serve immediately.

PER SERVING: Calories: 241 | Fat: 4g | Protein: 30g | Sodium: 103mg | Fiber: 3g | Carbohydrates: 22g | Sugar: 19g

Peaches and Cream Smoothie

A smoothie that supplies naturally occurring carbs from fruit with very low fat.

INGREDIENTS | SERVES 1

1 scoop vanilla protein powder
½ cup plain nonfat Greek yogurt
1 cup cold water
1 cup frozen peach chunks
Pinch stevia

Combine all ingredients in a blender and process until smooth. Serve immediately.

PER SERVING: Calories: 239 | Fat: 5g | Protein: 31g | Sodium: 103mg | Fiber: 2g | Carbohydrates: 21g | Sugar: 20g

Protein Piña Colada

This delicious, nonalcoholic take on a popular adult beverage is incredibly refreshing and easy to make.

INGREDIENTS | SERVES 1

1 scoop vanilla protein powder
½ cup frozen pineapple chunks
1 teaspoon coconut extract
½ cup skim milk
½ cup water
¼ cup shredded coconut
5 ice cubes

Combine all ingredients in a blender and process until smooth. Serve immediately.

PER SERVING: Calories: 268 | Fat: 8g | Protein: 30g | Sodium: 102mg | Fiber: 3g | Carbohydrates: 21g | Sugar: 17g

Peanut Butter and Jelly Smoothie

It may not sound terribly appealing, but this shake is delicious and has healthy fats to keep you full.

INGREDIENTS | SERVES 1

1 scoop vanilla protein powder
⅓ cup plain nonfat Greek yogurt
½ cup water
2 tablespoons natural peanut butter
½ cup frozen mixed berries
5 ice cubes

Combine all ingredients in a blender and process until smooth. Serve immediately.

PER SERVING: Calories: 386 | Fat: 19g | Protein: 36g | Sodium: 229mg | Fiber: 4g | Carbohydrates: 22g | Sugar: 15g

Tiramisu Smoothie

Here you get the flavors of the sinful Italian dessert without the excessive calories. This is the ultimate protein-filled shake for your enjoyment.

INGREDIENTS | SERVES 1

1 scoop chocolate protein powder
½ cup cottage cheese
1½ tablespoons slivered almonds
½ teaspoon instant coffee
Pinch stevia
5 ice cubes

Combine all ingredients in a blender and process until smooth. Serve immediately.

PER SERVING: Calories: 455 | Fat: 9g | Protein: 46g | Sodium: 443mg | Fiber: 1g | Carbohydrates: 46g | Sugar: 4g

Chocolate Peanut Butter Cup Smoothie

This smoothie has higher levels of fat and carbohydrates, making it suitable to be used as a meal replacement.

INGREDIENTS | SERVES 1

1 scoop chocolate protein powder
2 tablespoons natural peanut butter
1 tablespoon chocolate syrup
1 cup skim milk
Pinch stevia
5 ice cubes

Combine all ingredients in a blender and process until smooth. Serve immediately.

PER SERVING: Calories: 451 | Fat: 19g | Protein: 41g | Sodium: 309mg | Fiber: 2g | Carbohydrates: 32g | Sugar: 26g

Tropical Blend Smoothie

High carbs and high protein make this perfect for after a workout. It also has a lot of electrolytes from the fruit, so will help you stay hydrated on hot days.

INGREDIENTS | SERVES 1

1 scoop vanilla protein powder
1 medium banana
½ cup fresh pineapple
½ cup orange juice
½ cup pineapple juice
Pinch stevia
5 ice cubes

Combine all ingredients in a blender and process until smooth. Serve immediately.

PER SERVING: Calories: 378 | Fat: 1g | Protein: 28g | Sodium: 47mg | Fiber: 5g | Carbohydrates: 69g | Sugar: 46g

Pumpkin Pie Protein Shake

The perfect fall shake, this dessert-like concoction tastes like pumpkin pie in a glass. You could also top this with fat-free whipped cream for an extra treat.

INGREDIENTS | SERVES 1

1 scoop vanilla protein powder
½ cup canned pumpkin
1 cup almond milk
¼ cup crumbled graham cracker
1 teaspoon cinnamon
1 teaspoon nutmeg
Pinch stevia
5 ice cubes

Combine all ingredients in a blender and process until smooth. Serve immediately.

PER SERVING: Calories: 342 | Fat: 8g | Protein: 34g | Sodium: 296mg | Fiber: 6g | Carbohydrates: 34g | Sugar: 13g

Super Greens Shake

This is your ultimate meal replacement: It is loaded with protein, some carbs, healthy fats, and plenty of greens for antioxidants. You won't taste the greens, but they will be there supporting your overall health.

INGREDIENTS | SERVES 1

1 scoop chocolate protein powder

2 cups raw spinach

1 cup mixed berries

1 cup cold water

1 tablespoon natural peanut butter

Pinch stevia

5 ice cubes

Combine all ingredients in a blender and process until smooth. Serve immediately.

PER SERVING: Calories: 297 | Fat: 9g | Protein: 32g | Sodium: 170mg | Fiber: 6g | Carbohydrates: 28g | Sugar: 17g

CHAPTER 19

Desserts

Peanut Butter Protein Cookies
250

Oatmeal Protein Cookies
250

Protein Cheesecake
251

Peanut Butter Banana Frozen
Greek Yogurt
251

Frozen Chocolate Banana
252

Chocolate Banana Cups
253

No-Bake Cookie Bites
254

Mixed Berry Frozen Yogurt
255

Chocolate Pudding
255

Vanilla-Peach Dessert Bars
256

Double Chocolate Protein
Cookies
257

Cinnamon-Pear Frozen Yogurt
257

Fruit Salad
258

Cinnamon Pecan Cookie Bites
259

Peanut Butter Protein Cookies

The protein and fat in this recipe will keep you full with minimal carbohydrates. This is a perfect treat for low-carb days.

INGREDIENTS | SERVES 10

1 cup peanut butter
2 large egg whites
1 scoop vanilla protein powder
¾ cup stevia
1 teaspoon cinnamon

1. Preheat oven to 350°F.

2. Place all ingredients in a medium bowl and stir to combine.

3. Shape dough into 2" balls and place on greased cookie sheet.

4. Bake 10 minutes.

PER SERVING: Calories: 192 | Fat: 13g | Protein: 10g | Sodium: 133mg | Fiber: 2g | Carbohydrates: 12g | Sugar: 10g

Oatmeal Protein Cookies

These cookies are higher in carbs and protein with very low fat. The oatmeal also provides fiber, which will help keep you feeling full.

INGREDIENTS | SERVES 7

1¾ cup oats
4 scoops vanilla protein powder
½ cup applesauce
½ cup egg whites
1 tablespoon olive oil
1 tablespoon stevia
Dash cinnamon

1. Preheat oven to 350°F.

2. Place all ingredients in a large bowl and stir to mix.

3. Shape dough into 2" balls, and place on greased cookie sheet.

4. Bake 10–15 minutes.

PER SERVING: Calories: 170 | Fat: 3g | Protein: 19g | Sodium: 53mg | Fiber: 2g | Carbohydrates: 17g | Sugar: 3g

Protein Cheesecake

This recipe can be modified with any fruit or toppings you want to add, but stands fine on its own. Use fat-free cream cheese to keep calories in check.

INGREDIENTS | SERVES 8

24 ounces fat-free cream cheese
2 scoops vanilla whey protein powder
¾ cup stevia
1 teaspoon vanilla extract
3 large whole eggs
1 tablespoon lemon juice

1. Preheat oven to 350°F.

2. Place all ingredients in a large bowl and mix with hand mixer.

3. Pour mixture into a pie pan coated with nonstick cooking spray.

4. Bake 45 minutes. Remove from oven and refrigerate 3 hours or until ready to serve.

PER SERVING: Calories: 137 | Fat: 4g | Protein: 20g | Sodium: 501mg | Fiber: 0g | Carbohydrates: 5g | Sugar: 3g

Peanut Butter Banana Frozen Greek Yogurt

This dish is very quick to prepare and makes a well-rounded dessert that contains protein, carbs, and fat.

INGREDIENTS | SERVES 1

½ cup nonfat plain Greek yogurt
1 medium frozen banana, sliced
2 tablespoons peanut butter

Blend all ingredients in blender or food processor until smooth, and serve immediately.

PER SERVING: Calories: 342 | Fat: 17g | Protein: 14g | Sodium: 215mg | Fiber: 5g | Carbohydrates: 42g | Sugar: 26g

Frozen Chocolate Banana

The perfect summer treat, quick to prepare and easy to grab and enjoy.

INGREDIENTS | SERVES 2

2 medium bananas

4 ounces dark chocolate

½ cup ground peanuts, or any topping you prefer

Bananas for Exercise

When you are very active, especially during the summer months, it's very important to stay hydrated, as you can sweat out electrolytes. Bananas are not only a great source of natural sugar, they are full of potassium to keep you hydrated and help prevent cramping.

1. Peel bananas, cut in half, and place in freezer until firm.

2. Melt dark chocolate in a bowl in the microwave 3–5 minutes or until soft, or over the stove until soft.

3. Remove bananas from freezer and roll them in melted chocolate to cover, sprinkle with nuts or topping of choice, and return to the freezer until ready to enjoy.

PER SERVING: Calories: 290 | Fat: 17g | Protein: 7g | Sodium: 7mg | Fiber: 5g | Carbohydrates: 34g | Sugar: 23g

Chocolate Banana Cups

Just three ingredients come together to create this mouthwatering dessert that is a great source of carbs.

INGREDIENTS | SERVES 8

½ cup chocolate chips
¼ cup almond milk
1 medium banana, mashed

1. In a small saucepan over medium-low heat, melt chocolate chips and almond milk together until soft.

2. Once melted, pour a small amount into the bottom of some lined mini-muffin cups, just enough to cover the bottom of the cups. This recipe should fill 8 mini cups, but may vary depending on the size you are using.

3. Place muffin tin in the freezer 5–10 minutes.

4. Remove muffin tin and add a bit of mashed banana to each cup.

5. Fill cups with remaining amount of chocolate, and return to freezer until ready to serve.

PER SERVING: Calories: 88 | Fat: 4g | Protein: 1g | Sodium: 3mg | Fiber: 1g | Carbohydrates: 13g | Sugar: 9g

No-Bake Cookie Bites

This recipe uses alternative ingredients to make a healthy version of everyone's favorite dessert, chocolate chip cookies. It has good amounts of natural fats, carbs, and fiber, so it will fill you up.

INGREDIENTS | SERVES 8

1 cup oats
1 cup raw almonds
10–12 Medjool dates, pitted
½ cup water
¼ cup chocolate chips

1. Blend oats and almonds in a food processor until they become a powder.

2. Add dates, and continue to blend until well mixed.

3. Continue to blend while slowly adding water, until a thick paste texture forms.

4. Stir in chocolate chips, then roll mixture into bite-sized portions, place on lined baking sheet, and refrigerate until ready to serve.

PER SERVING: Calories: 172 | Fat: 8g | Protein: 4g | Sodium: 2mg | Fiber: 4g | Carbohydrates: 22g | Sugar: 11g

Mixed Berry Frozen Yogurt

This is a perfect high-carb-day snack—it is high in protein, low in fat, and with natural carbs and plenty of antioxidants.

INGREDIENTS | SERVES 1

½ cup nonfat plain Greek yogurt

1 cup frozen mixed berries

1 scoop protein powder, vanilla or chocolate

Blend all ingredients in a blender until smooth. Serve immediately.

PER SERVING: Calories: 264 | Fat: 5g | Protein: 30g | Sodium: 99mg | Fiber: 4g | Carbohydrates: 28g | Sugar: 21g

Chocolate Pudding

This pudding is ready in minutes, delicious, and full of protein, carbs, and fat to keep you full.

INGREDIENTS | SERVES 1

1¼ cups prepared chocolate pudding

1 scoop chocolate protein powder

1½ tablespoons coconut flakes

¼ cup fat-free whipped cream

Mix all ingredients except whipped cream in a medium bowl. Top with whipped cream and serve.

PER SERVING: Calories: 502 | Fat: 27g | Protein: 29g | Sodium: 95mg | Fiber: 7g | Carbohydrates: 15g | Sugar: 4g

Vanilla-Peach Dessert Bars

These sweet and delicious bars provide protein, carbs, and fiber and are very low fat.

INGREDIENTS | SERVES 4

¾ cup rolled oats

¼ cup oat bran

6 large egg whites

1 scoop vanilla protein powder

¼ teaspoon baking powder

¼ teaspoon stevia

Drop vanilla extract

2 medium peaches, peeled and diced

1. Preheat oven to 350°F.

2. Place all ingredients except peaches in a blender and blend until smooth. Transfer mixture to a medium bowl.

3. Add peaches to the mix and stir to combine.

4. Pour the mixture into a 9" × 9" baking dish, and bake 30 minutes. Cut into bars once cooled.

PER SERVING: Calories: 151 | Fat: 2g | Protein: 15g | Sodium: 123mg | Fiber: 4g | Carbohydrates: 22g | Sugar: 7g

Double Chocolate Protein Cookies

This rich and filling dessert is made with natural ingredients and no added sugar.

INGREDIENTS | SERVES 12

1 (15-ounce) can chickpeas, drained and rinsed

3 tablespoons water

⅓ cup chocolate protein powder

¾ cup chocolate chunks

1. Preheat oven to 350°F.

2. Add all ingredients except chocolate chunks to a blender and blend, adding water until it forms a thick dough.

3. Transfer mixture to a medium bowl and add chocolate chunks. Stir by hand to combine.

4. Form into golf ball–sized balls, place on greased cookie sheet, and bake 15 minutes.

PER SERVING: Calories: 121 | Fat: 4g | Protein: 5g | Sodium: 7mg | Fiber: 4g | Carbohydrates: 18g | Sugar: 8g

Cinnamon-Pear Frozen Yogurt

This delicious, fall-inspired frozen yogurt is high in carbs, and makes the perfect dessert for your high-carbohydrate days.

INGREDIENTS | SERVES 2

1 (15-ounce) can pear halves

2 cups low-fat vanilla yogurt

2 tablespoons stevia

½ teaspoon cinnamon

¼ teaspoon allspice

1. Drain pears, saving ½ cup of the juice.

2. Place pears in a blender or food processor and purée.

3. Add remaining ingredients and reserved pear juice to blender, blend until smooth, and freeze until ready to serve. You can also add the ingredients to an ice cream maker if you have one.

PER SERVING: Calories: 365 | Fat: 3g | Protein: 13g | Sodium: 172mg | Fiber: 6g | Carbohydrates: 74g | Sugar: 68g

Fruit Salad

This light and refreshing dessert is a great source of natural sugar and micronutrients. You can use any fruit you prefer; get creative.

INGREDIENTS | SERVES 4

2 cups sliced strawberries

1 pound seedless grapes, halved

3 medium bananas, peeled and sliced

1 (8-ounce) container low-fat strawberry yogurt

Mix all ingredients together in a large bowl, and chill until ready to serve.

PER SERVING: Calories: 234 | Fat: 1g | Protein: 4g | Sodium: 34mg | Fiber: 5g | Carbohydrates: 56g | Sugar: 42g

Get Some Fruit Variety

When consuming fruits and vegetables, you should try to get as much variety as possible, particularly in colors. Different colors will be higher in different micronutrients, which are the vitamins and minerals humans need for optimal health. Green, red, yellow, orange—eat as many colors as you can, rotating your sources on a regular basis. This will help you get all of your micronutrients and antioxidants.

Cinnamon Pecan Cookie Bites

Minimal ingredients provide a great source of healthy fats, and are very easy to prepare.

INGREDIENTS | SERVES 10

10 pitted dates, soaked in water 15 minutes

2 cups raw pecans

2 teaspoons cinnamon

1. Preheat oven to 350°F.

2. Drain dates, then combine all ingredients in food processor, blending until smooth.

3. Shape mixture into small balls and place on baking sheets lined with parchment paper.

4. Bake 10–12 minutes. Allow to cool before serving.

PER SERVING: Calories: 175 | Fat: 157g | Protein: 22g | Sodium: 2mg | Fiber: 30g | Carbohydrates: 96g | Sugar: 61g

Sample Menu Plan for High-Carb and Low-Carb Days

In the following lists, you'll see high- and low-carb options, with three and four meals each. The three-meal option would generally be for someone who is not working out, or for a rest day. The four-meal option would be for a strength-training day, with the fourth meal being a post-workout recovery meal.

Of course, you can always eat two meals per day, five meals per day, or any other number—these are just sample menus. On non-training days, you can eat your carbs whenever you want. On training days, try to keep at least half of them around your workout.

On any of the days, one or two small snacks may be added if you get hungry, or you can just eat larger meals.

High-Carb Day—3 Meals	
Meal 1	½ cup oats with sliced banana, 1 ounce almonds, and cinnamon, with side of 3 egg whites; coffee
Meal 2	Chicken Nachos (see Chapter 7)
Meal 3	Pulled Chicken BBQ Sandwich (see Chapter 7)
High-Carb Day—4 Meals	
Meal 1	Protein Scramble Bowl (see Chapter 6)
Meal 2	Slow-Cooked Chicken, shredded (see Chapter 7), and Homemade Buffalo Wing Sauce (see Chapter 14), with side of jasmine rice
Meal 3 (Post-workout)	Healthy Fried Rice (see Chapter 7), with side of a whey protein shake
Meal 4	Sirloin Chopped Salad (see Chapter 7), with piece of fruit
Low-Carb Day—3 Meals	
Meal 1	Protein Scramble Bowl (see Chapter 6)
Meal 2	Lemon-Herb Grilled Chicken Salad (see Chapter 7), with side of a handful of nuts
Meal 3	6 ounces salmon, with side of 2 cups of steamed vegetables with butter; glass of red wine
Low-Carb Day—4 Meals	
Meal 1	Greek Egg Scramble (see Chapter 6)
Meal 2	Tuna Salad (see Chapter 7), with side of a handful of berries and nuts
Meal 3 (Post-workout)	Low-Fat Chicken Bacon Ranch Sandwich (see Chapter 7), with side of a piece of fruit
Meal 4	Argentinian Steak (see Chapter 8), with side of steamed vegetables

As you can see, even on low-carb days, you still want some carbs after your workout to aid recovery. Even if you are only eating a small amount, such as 75 grams per day, try to put most of them around your workout.

Best Food Sources for Each Macronutrient Group

These are the best sources of each macronutrient, chosen because they are generally nutritious whole-food options. If your grocery list is mostly made up of items on this list, you are all set. There are other good foods that are not represented on this list, but these mentioned are the most readily available ones.

Plenty of foods would be considered "hybrids," such as a whole egg, which is nearly equal parts protein and fat, fatty cuts of meat, or processed foods that are high in carbs and fat. Those foods will be listed at the end, on their own separate list, as they are hard to classify under just one macronutrient.

Protein	Fat
Boneless, skinless chicken breast	Avocado
Egg whites	Cooking oils
Extra-lean ground beef	Grass-fed butter
Lean cuts red meat	Nut butter
Lean turkey breast/ground turkey	
Low-fat fish (such as tilapia, cod, or canned tuna)	
Nonfat cottage cheese	
Pork chops	
Whey protein powder	

Carbohydrates	Hybrids
Fruit	Cheese
Oatmeal, unflavored	Fatty cuts of fish
Pasta	Greek yogurt
Potatoes, any kind	Turkey bacon
Rice, any kind	Whole eggs
Whole-grain toast	

APPENDIX C

FAQ

Q: Should I be taking any supplements?

A: By definition, supplements only add to what you already have in place. It's best to try to get the majority of your nutrition from whole food sources, as it's impossible to supplement your way to good health with a bad diet.

There are a select few supplements that may be useful to add if your diet is on point, such as fish oil, vitamin D, creatine, and possibly a greens powder. For more information on when they may be appropriate, and specific product recommendations, visit *www.theathleticphysique.com/carb-cycling-book*.

Q: How should I track alcohol intake?

A: Alcohol is tricky. It has 7 calories per gram, but it provides no nutritional value—the definition of empty calories. Drinking in moderation is acceptable, but be aware that you'll have to make sacrifices elsewhere.

Liquor and dry wine can be counted as roughly 100 calories per serving. If you add mixers, or drink beer, the nutritional content can range all over the place. Regardless, if you are going to drink and want to stay within your caloric limits for the day, subtract the calories of your alcohol from your carb and/or fat total calories for the day. You should still try to get your daily protein in, but you can take calories from carbs and fat to drink alcohol.

Q: Can I really eat processed, sugary foods on this plan?

A: Yes. All things considered, your body doesn't discriminate against any specific food. Energy is energy—it's the laws of physics. From a nutritional value, of course there is a difference between oatmeal with fresh fruit and, say, a doughnut. You should aim to eat as much nutritious food as possible to optimize your health. However, if you really want to eat a sweet, as long as calories are the same, it won't make a difference when it comes to body composition. You could theoretically get all of your calories from processed food and still see results; you just wouldn't feel as good as you would eating nutritious food.

Q: How long will it take me to reach my goal?

A: This is a tough question. In general, you should aim for 1–2 pounds of fat loss per week. However, life happens, and so this exact amount of weight loss may not always occur. You can't say exactly that you'll lose 24 pounds in 12 weeks, for example. It might happen, but it might not.

To be conservative and allow for social events, minor slip-ups, and daily life, you can probably assume 5 pounds of fat lost per month, assuming you are sticking with the program at least 90 percent of the time.

While on this topic, it's important to realize that fat loss won't always be linear. If you use a scale to track progress, it's best to only weigh yourself once per week. Daily fluctuations can be caused by a variety of factors, and watching your weight move up and down every day can be discouraging. You want long-term results, with a downward trend in body weight. No need to get worried if your weight goes up or down by a pound or two; look at the long-term trend.

Q: What if I get stuck?

A: If you get stuck and can't lose fat while carb cycling, have a look at what you currently do. If you've just started, try to see if you can get more precise with your tracking, or implement one of the advanced strategies in Chapter 4.

If you've been doing this for a while, have your nutrition dialed in, and are exercising regularly, then it just comes down to creating a greater caloric deficit. You can either eat less or burn more calories. If you find your weight has been stuck for at least 10 days, and you've been consistent and accurate, start by removing around 200 calories from your daily intake, from a combination of carbs and fat.

If you prefer to eat more, you can also add more weekly cardio. Start by adding an additional 30-minute, moderate-intensity activity such as a jog or bike ride, and see what happens. You always have the choice between eating less or moving more—it's all personal preference.

Additional Resources

www.theathleticphysique.com/carb-cycling-book
A page on the author's website specifically for this book.
Features workout demonstration photos, links to specific product
recommendations, a FAQ that will be updated as questions come in, and
more bonus features for the book.

www.examine.com
Unbiased, extremely comprehensive research review of nearly
every supplement ingredient available. If you're considering taking a
supplement, check it out on Examine.com first.

Standard U.S./Metric Measurement Conversions

VOLUME CONVERSIONS

U.S. Volume Measure	Metric Equivalent
⅛ teaspoon	0.5 milliliter
¼ teaspoon	1 milliliter
½ teaspoon	2 milliliters
1 teaspoon	5 milliliters
½ tablespoon	7 milliliters
1 tablespoon (3 teaspoons)	15 milliliters
2 tablespoons (1 fluid ounce)	30 milliliters
¼ cup (4 tablespoons)	60 milliliters
⅓ cup	80 milliliters
½ cup (4 fluid ounces)	125 milliliters
⅔ cup	160 milliliters
¾ cup (6 fluid ounces)	180 milliliters
1 cup (16 tablespoons)	250 milliliters
1 pint (2 cups)	500 milliliters
1 quart (4 cups)	1 liter (about)

WEIGHT CONVERSIONS

U.S. Weight Measure	Metric Equivalent
½ ounce	15 grams
1 ounce	30 grams
2 ounces	60 grams
3 ounces	85 grams
¼ pound (4 ounces)	115 grams
½ pound (8 ounces)	225 grams
¾ pound (12 ounces)	340 grams
1 pound (16 ounces)	454 grams

OVEN TEMPERATURE CONVERSIONS

Degrees Fahrenheit	Degrees Celsius
200 degrees F	95 degrees C
250 degrees F	120 degrees C
275 degrees F	135 degrees C
300 degrees F	150 degrees C
325 degrees F	160 degrees C
350 degrees F	180 degrees C
375 degrees F	190 degrees C
400 degrees F	205 degrees C
425 degrees F	220 degrees C
450 degrees F	230 degrees C

BAKING PAN SIZES

American	Metric
8 × 1½ inch round baking pan	20 × 4 cm cake tin
9 × 1½ inch round baking pan	23 × 3.5 cm cake tin
11 × 7 × 1½ inch baking pan	28 × 18 × 4 cm baking tin
13 × 9 × 2 inch baking pan	30 × 20 × 5 cm baking tin
2 quart rectangular baking dish	30 × 20 × 3 cm baking tin
15 × 10 × 2 inch baking pan	38 × 25 × 5 cm baking tin (Swiss roll tin)
9 inch pie plate	22 × 4 or 23 × 4 cm pie plate
7 or 8 inch springform pan	18 or 20 cm springform or loose bottom cake tin
9 × 5 × 3 inch loaf pan	23 × 13 × 7 cm or 2 lb narrow loaf or pate tin
1½ quart casserole	1.5 liter casserole
2 quart casserole	2 liter casserole

Index

Note: Page numbers in **bold** indicate recipe category lists.

Adobo Seasoning, 184
Alcohol, 14, 270
Almonds, sweet and spicy, 235
Anti-inflammatory foods, 82, 120
Antioxidants, functions of, 18
Antioxidants, sources of, 78, 79, 146, 156, 227, 234, 235, 258
Apples
    about: hunger-fighting effects of, 208
    Apple, Pear, and Cranberry Crisp with Fresh Ginger, 236
    Apple Cinnamon Oatmeal, 72
    Apple Coleslaw, 147
    Butternut Squash and Apple Fall Soup, 177
    Cinnamon Apple Snack Bars, 211
    Cinnamon Protein Apple Slices, 212
    No-Bake Apple Crisp, 208
    Pork Loin with Baked Apples, 220
Argentinian Steak, 108
    Artichoke and Olive Pasta, 160
Asparagus, pickled, 197
Asparagus Salad with Hard-Boiled Egg, 99
Avocados
    about: fats from, 120
    Fresh Salsa, 80
    Power Wrap, 72
    Protein Guacamole, 213

Bacon
    Egg White Protein Bites, 74

Low-Calorie Bacon, Egg, and Cheese, 76
Low-Fat Chicken Bacon Ranch Sandwich, 89
Portobello Mushroom Salad with Gorgonzola, Peppers, and Bacon, 98
Power Wrap, 72
Baked Buffalo Chicken Strips, 102
Baked Eggplant and Bell Pepper, 131
Baked Ravioli, 158
Balsamic Vinaigrette, 182
Bananas
    about: for exercise, 252
    Banana Oatmeal, 129
    Banana Protein Pudding, 209
    Chocolate Banana Cups, 253
    Chocolate Banana Protein Pancakes, 71
    Frozen Chocolate Banana, 252
    Key Lime Pie Smoothie, 242
    Peanut Butter Banana Frozen Greek Yogurt, 251
    Tropical Blend Smoothie, 246
Barley, in Mushroom Barley Pilaf with Fresh Green Beans, 229
Basil Pesto. *See* Pesto
    Bean Salad with Orange Vinaigrette, 136
Beans and other legumes
    about: chickpea nutritional benefits and uses, 156
    Bean Salad with Orange Vinaigrette, 136
    Black Bean and King Oyster Mushroom Soup, 177
    Chicken and Bean Burrito, 104
    Corn and Black Bean Chili, 170

Double Chocolate Protein Cookies, 257
Garlicky Chickpeas and Spinach, 156
Lentil Salad, 97
Mediterranean Chickpea Bake, 144
Mini Vegetable Burgers, 145
Red Beans and Rice, 143
Shepherd's Pie, 223
Southwestern Omelet, 71
Spring Pea and Mint Soup, 175
Vegetarian Cakes, 128
Whole-Wheat Penne with Kale and Cannellini Beans, 159
Beef
    about: steak selection, 108
    Argentinian Steak, 108
    Dry Rub for Ribs, 189
    Lean Meat Balls, 109
    Pressure Cooker Beef Bourguignon, 219
    Sirloin Chopped Salad, 90
    Slow Cooker Beef Stew, 178
    Steakhouse Blue Cheese Burger, 109
Beer Can Chicken, 111
Beets, in Roasted Beet Celeriac Mash, 195
    Beets, in Southwestern Beet Slaw, 135
Beets, peeling easily, 195
Benefits of carb cycling, 25–34
    about: overview of, 25
    blood sugar stabilization, 28–29
    caloric deficit for fat loss, 31–34
    energy, 29–30
    enjoying foods you like, 34

Benefits of carb cycling—*continued*
    hormonal profile
        improvement, 31
    hunger control, 30–31
    mental clarity and focus, 29–30
Berries
    about: freezing cranberries, 236;
        nutritional benefits, 78, 210
    Apple, Pear, and Cranberry
        Crisp with Fresh Ginger, 236
    Berries and Cream Parfait, 78
    Blue Velvet Smoothie, 241
    Chocolate-Covered Berry
        Delight, 214
    Mixed Berry Frozen Yogurt, 255
    Neapolitan Smoothie, 241
    Peanut Butter and Jelly
        Smoothie, 244
    Protein Sludge, 215
    Super Greens Shake, 247
    Triple Berry Parfait, 210
    Two-Minute Chocolate
        Strawberry Protein Bowl, 75
    Vanilla Raspberry Protein
        Fluff, 77
Beverages. *See* Drinks
Biscuits, buttermilk, 231
Black beans. *See* Beans and
    other legumes
Blackberries and blueberries.
    See Berries
Blood sugar
    absorption into bloodstream, 26
    diabetes and, 26, 27
    fruit, vegetables and, 28
    high carbohydrate intake
        impact, 27–28
    importance of monitoring, 26
    insulin sensitivity and, 27, 28
    stabilizing, 28–29
Blue Velvet Smoothie, 241
Book overview, 11–12, 66–68
Breads
    about: best for sandwiches,
        89. *See also* Sandwiches
        and wraps
    Buttermilk Biscuits, 231

    Red Onion and Olive
        Focaccia, 153
Breakfast, **69**–83
    about: boosting fiber with, 76;
        complete protein snacks, 74;
        protein made easy, 73
    Apple Cinnamon Oatmeal, 72
    Berries and Cream Parfait, 78
    Chocolate Banana Protein
        Pancakes, 71
    Clean Protein Power Bars, 82
    Egg White Protein Bites, 74
    Greek Egg Scramble, 70
    High-Protein French Toast, 73
    Homemade Scallion Hash
        Brown Cakes, 83
    Huevos Rancheros, 80
    Low-Calorie Bacon, Egg, and
        Cheese, 76
    Power Wrap, 72
    Protein Scramble Bowl, 75
    Simple Sweet Potato
        Pancakes, 81
    Southwestern Omelet, 71
    Spinach, Red Onion, and
        Mushroom Frittata, 79
    Two-Minute Chocolate
        Strawberry Protein Bowl, 75
    Vanilla Raspberry Protein
        Fluff, 77
Broccoli
    Broccoli-Basil Pesto and
        Pasta, 161
    Broccoli-Cauliflower Bake, 203
    Chicken and Broccoli
    Fettuccine, 162
    Cream of Broccoli Soup, 180
    Quinoa with Mixed
        Vegetables, 202
    Broccoli-Basil Pesto and
        Pasta, 161
Brussels sprouts, roasted radishes
    and, 224
Brussels sprouts, sweet and
    spicy, 155
Buffalo Chicken Macaroni and
    Cheese, 165

Buffalo wing sauce,
    homemade, 188
Burgers. *See* Sandwiches
    and wraps
Burritos, chicken and bean, 104
Burritos, quinoa, 104
Buttermilk Biscuits, 231
Butternut squash. *See* Squash
Buttery Garlic Pasta, 165

Cabbage
    Apple Coleslaw, 147
    Portobello Tacos, 139
Cajun Seasoning, 185
Calories
    alcohol and, 14, 270
    calculating total intake, 38, 40
    counting with carb
        cycling, 23–24
    deficit, for fat loss, 31–34
    determining intake levels, 37–41
    fiber and, 19–20
    key to fat loss, 22–23
    macronutrient conversion
        rates, 39
    reverse dieting
        importance, 61–63
    sources of, 14–15, 265–67
Canning fruits and vegetables, 197
Carb back-loading, 57–58
Carb cycling. *See also*
    Carbohydrates; High-carb days;
    Low-carb days
    advanced. *See* Carb cycling,
        advanced strategies
    around workouts, 54–55. *See
        also* Exercise
    basic form of, 21–22
    breaking through plateaus,
        55–58, 271
    duration of use, 60, 63–64. *See
        also* Maintenance phase
    FAQ, 269–71
    instinctive eating vs., 64–65
    multilevel, 56
    starting out. *See* Carb cycling,
        getting started

this book and, 11–12, 66–68
time to reach fat-loss goals, 271
weekly depletion and
    re-feed, 56–57
what it is, 13, 20
what it is not, 20
Carb cycling, advanced
    strategies, 47–58
about: overview of, 47
adding exercise, 48
endurance (cardio) and
    strength training, 49–55. *See
    also* Exercise
fat-loss plateau solutions, 55–58
Carb cycling, getting started
about: overview of, 35
adding green veggies to all
    meals, 45
"cheat" meal plans, 43–44
determining intake levels
    (calories, protein, carbs, and
    fats), 37–41
eating most carbs before/after
    workouts, 44
good and bad nutrient
    combos, 43
meal planning, 41–42
scheduling high- and low-carb
    days, 36–37
setting carb numbers, 40–41
tips, tricks to maximize
    results, 44–45
water intake and, 45
Carbohydrates. *See also Carb
cycling references*
balancing other macronutrients
    with, 15
breakdown of, 26
calculating daily needs, 39–40
calorie counting and.
    See Calories
calorie values, 14–15
eating most before/after
    workouts, 44
functions of, 15–16
glucose from. *See* Blood sugar
glycemic index and, 20

good and bad nutrient
    combos, 43
high-carb-day sources, 21
high intake problems, 27–28
"hybrid" foods and, 266
impact on body, 26
low-carb-day sources,
    21–22
as macronutrients, 14
sources of, 16–17, 18
Carrots
Roasted Root Vegetables with
    Orange and Thyme, 230
Sweet and Spicy Carrot
    Soup, 174
Vegetable Stew with Cornmeal
    Dumplings, 142
Cashew-Zucchini Soup, 151
Cauliflower
Broccoli-Cauliflower Bake, 203
Creamy Cauliflower Soup, 176
Shepherd's Pie, 223
Vegetable Stew with Cornmeal
    Dumplings, 142
Ceviche, shrimp, 125
Chard, rainbow, with farrow, 198
Chard, Swiss, and kohlrabi, 192
"Cheat" meal plans, 43–44
Cheese
about: goat cheese
    superiority, 203
Broccoli-Cauliflower Bake, 203
Crispy Parmesan Fish Sticks,
    123
eggs with. *See* Eggs
Feta and Tuna Pasta Salad, 123
Goat Cheese–Stuffed Dates, 234
High-Protein Spread, 128
Key Lime Pie Smoothie, 242
Nutty Cottage Cheese, 211
pasta with. *See* Pasta
Protein Cheesecake, 251
Protein Guacamole, 213
sandwiches/wraps with. *See*
    Sandwiches and wraps
Spinach and Feta Salmon, 119
Tiramisu Smoothie, 245

Chicken. *See Poultry references*
Chicken and Broccoli
    Fettuccine, 162
Chickpeas
about: nutritional benefits and
    uses, 156
Double Chocolate Protein
    Cookies, 257
Garlicky Chickpeas and
    Spinach, 156
Mediterranean Chickpea
    Bake, 144
Chili, corn and black bean, 170
Chocolate
Blue Velvet Smoothie, 241
Chocolate Banana Cups, 253
Chocolate Banana Protein
    Pancakes, 71
Chocolate-Covered Berry
    Delight, 214
Chocolate Peanut Butter Cup
    Smoothie, 245
Chocolate Pomegranate
    Brownies, 237
Chocolate Pudding, 255
Double Chocolate Protein
    Cookies, 257
Frozen Chocolate Banana, 252
Mint Chocolate Chip
    Smoothie, 242
Mocha Protein Bars, 209
Neapolitan Smoothie, 241
No-Bake Cookie Bites, 254
Tiramisu Smoothie, 245
Two-Minute Chocolate
    Strawberry Protein Bowl, 75
Cinnamon
Apple Cinnamon Oatmeal, 72
Cinnamon Apple Snack Bars, 211
Cinnamon Chai Latte
    Smoothie, 240
Cinnamon-Pear Frozen
    Yogurt, 257
Cinnamon Pecan Cookie
    Bites, 259
Cinnamon Protein Apple
    Slices, 212

Citrus
    about: benefits of lemon
      juice, 95
    Citrus Vinaigrette, 183
    Key Lime Pie Smoothie, 242
    Lemon and Garlic Cod
      Fillets, 122
    Lemon-Herb Grilled Chicken
      Salad, 95
    Lemon Pepper Tilapia, 124
    Lemon Quinoa, 133
    Orange Cream Delight, 243
    Orange-Sesame Dressing, 149
    Tropical Blend Smoothie, 246
Clean Protein Power Bars, 82
Coconut, in Protein Piña
    Colada, 244
Coconut Garlic Shrimp, 118
Cod fillets, 122
Coffee, in Mocha Protein Bars,
    209
Coffee, in Tiramisu Smoothie, 245
Coleslaw, apple, 147
Cookies. *See* Desserts
Corn
    Corn and Black Bean Chili, 170
    Creamy Corn Chowder, 171
    Fresh Corn, Pepper, and
      Avocado Salad, 134
    Sage-Parmesan Polenta, 199
    Vegetable Stew with Cornmeal
      Dumplings, 142
    Vegetable-Stuffed Poblano
      Peppers, 138
    Cream of Broccoli Soup, 180
Crispy Parmesan Fish Sticks, 123
Curry Seasoning, 186

Dates
    about: nutritional benefits, 234
    Cinnamon Pecan Cookie
      Bites, 259
    Goat Cheese–Stuffed Dates, 234
    No-Bake Cookie Bites, 254
Depletion, weekly re-feed
    and, 56–57
Desserts, **249**–59. *See also* Snacks

about: eating processed, sugary
    foods, 270
Apple, Pear, and Cranberry
    Crisp with Fresh Ginger, 236
Chocolate Banana Cups, 253
Chocolate Pomegranate
    Brownies, 237
Chocolate Pudding, 255
Cinnamon-Pear Frozen
    Yogurt, 257
Cinnamon Pecan Cookie
    Bites, 259
Double Chocolate Protein
    Cookies, 257
Frozen Chocolate Banana, 252
Fruit Salad, 258
Mixed Berry Frozen Yogurt, 255
No-Bake Cookie Bites, 254
Oatmeal Protein Cookies, 250
Peanut Butter Banana Frozen
    Greek Yogurt, 251
Peanut Butter Protein
    Cookies, 250
Pound Cake Minis, 238
Protein Cheesecake, 251
Vanilla-Peach Dessert Bars, 256
Diabetes, 26, 27
Diet. *See also* Carb cycling
references; Maintenance phase
    best food sources for
      macronutrients, 18–19, 265–67
    building caloric deficit
      with, 31–32
    building caloric deficit with
      exercise and, 33–34
    determining intake levels, 37–41
    eating out, 42
    enjoying foods you like, 34
    "hybrid" foods and, 266
    meal planning, 41–42
    reverse dieting
      importance, 61–63
Dijon Tuna, 118
Dinner, vegetarian. *See* Vegetarian
    mains, sides, and salads
Dinner: Beef, pork, and poultry,
    101–15. *See also* Holiday recipes

Argentinian Steak, 108
Baked Buffalo Chicken
    Strips, 102
Beer Can Chicken, 111
Chicken and Bean Burrito, 104
Garlic-Studded Pork Roast, 115
Lean Meat Balls, 109
Lean Turkey Meatloaf, 113
Marinated Grilled Turkey
    Cutlets, 114
Mustard Pecan Chicken, 106
Papaya Pulled Pork, 104
Pesto Pork Chops, 107
Spaghetti Marinara with Chicken
    and Basil, 112
Steakhouse Blue Cheese
    Burger, 109
Sun-Dried Tomato Stuffed
    Chicken, 103
Tamarind Pot Roast, 105
Tuscan Chicken, 110
Dinner: Fish and shellfish. *See* Fish
    and shellfish, dinner recipes
Dinner: Vegan and vegetarian.
    See Vegan mains, sides, and
    salads; Vegetarian mains, sides,
    and salads
Double Chocolate Protein
    Cookies, 257
Drinks, **239**–47
    about: protein powder for, 240
    Blue Velvet Smoothie, 241
    Chocolate Peanut Butter Cup
      Smoothie, 245
    Cinnamon Chai Latte
      Smoothie, 240
    Key Lime Pie Smoothie,
      242
    Mint Chocolate Chip
      Smoothie, 242
    Neapolitan Smoothie, 241
    Orange Cream Delight, 243
    Peaches and Cream
      Smoothie, 243
    Peanut Butter and Jelly
      Smoothie, 244
    Protein Piña Colada, 244

Pumpkin Pie Protein Shake, 246
Super Greens Shake, 247
Tiramisu Smoothie, 245
Tropical Blend Smoothie, 246
Dry Rub for Ribs, 189

Eating out, 42
Eggplant and bell pepper,
    baked, 131
Eggs
    about: hard boiling, 99, 212
    Asparagus Salad with Hard-
        Boiled Egg, 99
    Clean Protein Power Bars, 82
    Egg White Protein Bites, 74
    Greek Egg Scramble, 70
    Hard-Boiled Eggs, 212
    Herb Mashed Eggs, 213
    High-Protein French Toast, 73
    Huevos Rancheros, 80
    Low-Calorie Bacon, Egg, and
        Cheese, 76
    Power Wrap, 72
    Protein Scramble Bowl, 75
    Sausage and Spicy Eggs, 96
    Southwestern Eggs, 214
    Southwestern Omelet, 71
    Spinach, Red Onion, and
        Mushroom Frittata, 79
Endurance training. See Exercise
Exercise
    about: bananas for, 252
    adding, 48
    building caloric deficit with diet
        and, 32–34
    calories burned with, 33
    cycling carbs around
        workouts, 54–55
    eating most carbs before/
        after, 44
    endurance (cardio)
        program, 50–51
    endurance (cardio) vs. strength
        training, 49–50
    importance in losing fat, 48
    non-exercise activity (NEAT)
        and, 32

resistance training
    advantages, 37
    scheduling high-/low-carb days
        and, 36–37
    strength-training
        workouts, 51–54

Fajitas, 90
FAQ, 269–71
Farro with Rainbow Chard, 198
Fat loss (body fat)
    building caloric deficit for, 31–34
    carb back-loading for, 57–58
    food intake as key to, 22–23
    high-carb days without gaining
        fat and, 65–66
    mechanics of, 22–23
    multilevel carb cycling for, 56
    plateaus, breaking through,
        55–58, 271
    sweating and, 23
    time to reach goals, 271
    weekly depletion and re-feed
        for, 56–57
    working out for. See Exercise
Fats (dietary)
    balancing other macronutrients
        with, 15
    calculating daily needs, 39–40
    calorie values and, 14–15
    functions of, 15
    getting fat and, 15
    good and bad nutrient
        combos, 43
    high-carb days and, 21
    low-carb days and, 21–22
    as macronutrients, 14
    sources of, 17–18, 19, 267
Fennel
    about, 146
    Arugula and Fennel Salad with
        Pomegranate, 146
    Red Pepper and Fennel
        Salad, 150
Fettuccine. See Pasta
Fiber
    boosting with breakfast, 76

counting calories and, 19–20
    defined, 19
    supplements, 20
Fish and shellfish
    about: bad fats in, 120; fat
        content by type, 19; healthy
        fats in, 92, 120, 123
    Black Bean and King Oyster
        Mushroom Soup, 177
    Oyster Portobello
        Un-Stuffing, 226
    Pepper, Onion, and Shrimp
        Kebabs, 164
    Shrimp Noodles with Chinese
        Chives, 167
    Shrimp Orzo Salad, 163
    Shrimp Shiitake Pot Stickers, 233
    Shrimp Stir-Fry, 86
    Spaghetti Squash Crab Blend, 89
    Tuna Salad, 92
Fish and shellfish, dinner
    recipes, **117**–25
    about: leanest fish, 123; selecting
        fish, 118, 123; shrimp, 222;
        wild-caught vs. farm-raised
        salmon, 121
    Coconut Garlic Shrimp, 118
    Crispy Parmesan Fish Sticks, 123
    Dijon Tuna, 118
    Feta and Tuna Pasta Salad, 123
    High-Protein Tuna Melt, 124
    Lemon and Garlic Cod
        Fillets, 122
    Lemon Pepper Tilapia, 124
    Salmon Burgers, 120
    Shrimp Ceviche, 125
    Shrimp Creole, 222
    Shrimp-Orange Kebabs, 119
    Shrimp Scampi, 122
    Spinach and Feta Salmon, 119
    Stuffed Salmon Fillets, 121
    Sun-Dried Tomato Tuna, 121
Fluff, vanilla raspberry, 77
Focaccia, 153
Fondant Potatoes and Pearl
    Onions, 194
Free radicals, neutralizing, 18

French Dressing, 97
French toast, high-protein, 73
Frozen Chocolate Banana, 252
Fruits. *See also specific fruits*
    about: blood sugar and, 28;
        canning, 197; getting variety
        of, 258; nutritional benefits, 28
    Fruit Salad, 258

Garbanzo beans. *See* Chickpeas
Garlic
    about: uses and benefits, 115
    Buttery Garlic Pasta, 165
    Coconut Garlic Shrimp, 118
    Garlic Kale Chips, 216
    Garlicky Chickpeas and
        Spinach, 156
    Garlic Rosemary Mashed
        Potatoes, 227
    Garlic-Studded Pork Roast, 115
    Lemon and Garlic Cod
        Fillets, 122
Glucose. *See* Blood sugar
Glycemic index, 20
Greek Egg Scramble, 70
Green beans, mushroom barley
    pilaf with, 229
Grocery shopping, 42

Hard-Boiled Eggs, 99, 212
Healthy Fried Rice, 94
Herb Mashed Eggs, 213
Herbs and spices, 114, 143, 227,
    230. *See also* Sauces, dressings,
    and rubs
High-carb days
    explained, 21
    fat intake and, 21
    food sources for, 21, 267
    meal plans (3 or 4 meals), 263
    protein sources for, 21, 267
    scheduling, 36–37
    setting numbers for, 40–41
    without gaining fat
        (ongoing), 65–66
High-Protein Spread, 128
High-Protein Tuna Melt, 124

Holiday recipes, **217**–38
    Apple, Pear, and Cranberry
        Crisp with Fresh Ginger, 236
    Buttermilk Biscuits, 231
    Chocolate Pomegranate
        Brownies, 237
    Easy Dumpling Dipping
        Sauce, 233
    Garlic Rosemary Mashed
        Potatoes, 227
    Goat Cheese–Stuffed Dates, 234
    Mushroom Barley Pilaf with
        Fresh Green Beans, 229
    Oyster Portobello
        Un-Stuffing, 226
    Pork Loin with Baked
        Apples, 220
    Pound Cake Minis, 238
    Pressure Cooker Beef
        Bourguignon, 219
    Roasted Radishes and Brussels
        Sprouts, 224
    Roasted Root Vegetables with
        Orange and Thyme, 230
    Rosemary Wild Rice Pilaf, 232
    Shepherd's Pie, 223
    Shrimp Creole, 222
    Shrimp Shiitake Pot Stickers, 233
    Spice-Rubbed Roasted Turkey
        Breast, 218
    Sweet and Spicy Almonds, 235
    Vegetable Baked Ziti, 225
    Whipped Butternut Squash, 228
    Whipped Sweet Potatoes, 228
    Whole-Grain Rotini with Pork,
        Pumpkin, and Sage, 221
Homemade Buffalo Wing
    Sauce, 188
Homemade Scallion Hash Brown
    Cakes, 83
Hormonal profile, 31
Huevos Rancheros, 80
Hunger, controlling, 30–31, 208
Hydration, 45

Ingredients. *See also specific main
    ingredients*

best food sources for
    macronutrients, 18–19, 265–67
grocery shopping for, 42
meal planning and, 41–42
preparing, 42
profiles of, meal plans and, 182
Insulin sensitivity, 27

Kale
    Garlic Kale Chips, 216
    Kale and Sea Vegetables with
        Orange-Sesame Dressing, 149
    Spicy Peanut Tempeh Salad, 131
Key Lime Pie Smoothie, 242
Kohlrabi and Swiss Chard, 192

Lean Meat Balls, 109
Lean Turkey Meatloaf, 113
Lemon. *See* Citrus
Lentil Salad, 97
Low-Calorie Bacon, Egg, and
    Cheese, 76
Low-carb days
    explained, 21–22
    fat intake and, 21–22
    food sources for, 21, 267
    meal plans (3 or 4 meals), 263
    misconception about, 21
    scheduling, 36–37
    setting numbers for, 40–41
Lunch, **85**–99
    about: best sandwich bread, 89
    Asparagus Salad with Hard-
        Boiled Egg, 99
    Chicken Nachos, 93
    Healthy Fried Rice, 94
    Lemon-Herb Grilled Chicken
        Salad, 95
    Lentil Salad, 97
    Low-Fat Chicken Bacon Ranch
        Sandwich, 89
    Portobello Mushroom Salad with
        Gorgonzola, Peppers, and
        Bacon, 98
    Pulled Chicken BBQ
        Sandwich, 93
    Sausage and Spicy Eggs, 96

Shrimp Stir-Fry, 86
Sirloin Chopped Salad, 90
Slow-Cooked Chicken, 87
Southwestern Fajitas, 90
Spaghetti Squash Crab Blend, 89
Spinach, Feta, and Pesto
    Chicken Quesadillas, 91
Tuna Salad, 92
Turkey Burgers, 88

Macaroni and cheese, 165
Macronutrients. *See also*
    Carbohydrates; Fats
    (dietary); Proteins
    balancing, 15
    calorie conversion rates, 39
    calorie values and, 14–15
    defined, 14
    functions of, 15–16
    sources of, 16–19, 265–67
Main dishes. *See Dinner references*;
    Pasta; Vegan mains, sides, and
    salads; Vegetarian mains, sides,
    and salads
Maintenance phase, 59–68
    about: overview of, 59
    carb cycling duration and,
        60, 63–64
    high-carb days without gaining
        fat, 65–66
    instinctive eating vs. carb
        cycling, 64–65
    reverse dieting
        importance, 61–63
    transitioning to "normal" eating
        style, 61
Marinara Sauce, 112
Marinated Grilled Turkey
    Cutlets, 114
Meal plans. *See also* Ingredients;
    Recipes; *specific main
    ingredients*
    eating different foods for
        variety, 68
    guidelines for creating, 41–42, 68
    high-carb day (3 or 4 meals), 263
    ingredient profiles for, 182

low-carb day (3 or 4 meals), 263
    using plans in this book, 64,
        67–68, 262
Measurement conversions, 275
Meat balls, 109
Meatloaf, turkey, 113
Mediterranean Chickpea Bake, 144
Memphis seasoning, spicy, 186
Mental clarity and focus, 29–30
Metric conversions, 275
Mini Vegetable Burgers, 145
Mint
    Mint Chocolate Chip
        Smoothie, 242
    Spring Pea and Mint Soup, 175
Mint Chocolate Chip Smoothie, 242
Mixed Berry Frozen Yogurt, 255
Mocha Protein Bars, 209
Multilevel carb cycling, 56
Mushrooms
    about: portobellos, 139; types
        of, 98
    Black Bean and King Oyster
        Mushroom Soup, 177
    Mushroom Barley Pilaf with
        Fresh Green Beans, 229
    Oyster Portobello
        Un-Stuffing, 226
    Portobello Mushroom Salad with
        Gorgonzola, Peppers, and
        Bacon, 98
    Portobello Tacos, 139
    Quinoa with Mixed
        Vegetables, 202
    Shrimp Shiitake Pot Stickers, 233
    Spinach, Red Onion, and
        Mushroom Frittata, 79
    Stuffed Mushrooms, 204
    Ultimate Spinach and Mushroom
        Risotto, 201
Mustard Pecan Chicken, 106

Nachos, chicken, 93
Neapolitan Smoothie, 241
No-Bake Apple Crisp, 208
No-Bake Cookie Bites, 254
Noodles. *See* Pasta

Nutrients. *See* Carbohydrates;
    Fats (dietary); Macronutrients;
    Proteins; RDA
Nuts and seeds
    about: almond nutritional
        benefits, 235; flaxseed
        nutritional benefits, 82;
        nutritional differences
        between, 147; walnut oil,
        150
    Cashew-Zucchini Soup, 151
    Chocolate Peanut Butter Cup
        Smoothie, 245
    Cinnamon Pecan Cookie
        Bites, 259
    Clean Protein Power Bars, 82
    Mustard Pecan Chicken, 106
    No-Bake Cookie Bites, 254
    Nutty Cottage Cheese, 211
    Orange-Sesame Dressing, 149
    Peanut Butter and Jelly
        Smoothie, 244
    Peanut Butter Banana Frozen
        Greek Yogurt, 251
    Peanut Butter Protein
        Cookies, 250
    Spicy Peanut Tempeh Salad, 131
    Sweet and Spicy Almonds, 235

Oats
    about: as flour substitute, 71;
        using as is or blending into
        powder, 71
    Apple, Pear, and Cranberry
        Crisp with Fresh Ginger, 236
    Apple Cinnamon Oatmeal, 72
    Banana Oatmeal, 129
    Chocolate Banana Protein
        Pancakes, 71
    Cinnamon Apple Snack Bars, 211
    Clean Protein Power Bars, 82
    Mocha Protein Bars, 209
    No-Bake Cookie Bites, 254
    Oatmeal Protein Cookies, 250
    Vanilla-Peach Dessert Bars, 256
    Vegetarian Cakes, 128
Oils, 144, 150, 220

Olives
  about: making olive oil spray, 144, 220
  Red Onion and Olive Focaccia, 153
Onions
  about: using shallots instead of, 192
  Fondant Potatoes and Pearl Onions, 194
  Homemade Scallion Hash Brown Cakes, 83
  Red Onion and Olive Focaccia, 153
  Spinach, Red Onion, and Mushroom Frittata, 79
  Summer Vegetable Tian, 154
Orange. See Citrus
Oriental Seasoning, 187
Oven fries, zucchini, 132
Oyster Portobello Un-Stuffing, 226

Pancakes, chocolate banana protein, 71
Pancakes, sweet potato, 81
Papaya Pulled Pork, 104
Parfait, berries and cream, 78
Parfait, triple berry, 210
Parsnips, 148, 230
Pasta, **157**–67
  about: high-protein, 164; nutrient-enriched varieties, 164
  Artichoke and Olive Pasta, 160
  Baked Ravioli, 158
  Broccoli-Basil Pesto and Pasta, 161
  Buffalo Chicken Macaroni and Cheese, 165
  Buttery Garlic Pasta, 165
  Chicken and Broccoli Fettuccine, 162
  Chicken Ramen Soup, 179
  Farfalle with Chicken and Pesto, 158
  Feta and Tuna Pasta Salad, 123
  High-Protein Spaghetti, 164

Pasta with Ricotta and Lemon, 163
Shrimp Noodles with Chinese Chives, 167
Shrimp Orzo Salad, 163
Spaghetti Marinara with Chicken and Basil, 112
Tricolor Penne, 166
Vegetable Baked Ziti, 225
Whole-Grain Rotini with Pork, Pumpkin, and Sage, 221
Whole-Wheat Penne with Kale and Cannellini Beans, 159
Peaches, in Vanilla-Peach Dessert Bars, 256
Peaches and Cream Smoothie, 243
Peanut butter. See Nuts and seeds
Pears
  Apple, Pear, and Cranberry Crisp with Fresh Ginger, 236
  Cinnamon-Pear Frozen Yogurt, 257
  Vanilla Pear Vinaigrette, 184
Pecans. See Nuts and seeds
Pepper, Onion, and Shrimp Kebabs, 164
Peppers
  Baked Eggplant and Bell Pepper, 131
  Pepper, Onion, and Shrimp Kebabs, 164
  Portobello Mushroom Salad with Gorgonzola, Peppers, and Bacon, 98
  Red Pepper and Fennel Salad, 150
  Tuscan Chicken, 110
  Vegetable-Stuffed Poblano Peppers, 138
Pesto
  about: making, 91
  Basil Pesto, 187
  Broccoli-Basil Pesto and Pasta, 161
  Farfalle with Chicken and Pesto, 158

Pesto Pork Chops, 107
Spinach, Feta, and Pesto Chicken Quesadillas, 91
Pickled Asparagus, 197
Pineapple, in Protein Piña Colada, 244
Pineapple, in Tropical Blend Smoothie, 246
Plateaus, breaking through, 55–58, 271
Polenta, sage-Parmesan, 199
Pomegranate, arugula and fennel salad with, 146
Pomegranate, in Chocolate Pomegranate Brownies, 237
Pork
  Dry Rub for Ribs, 189
  Garlic-Studded Pork Roast, 115
  Chili Lime Pork Strips, 104
  Papaya Pulled Pork, 104
  Pork Loin with Baked Apples, 220
  Portobello Mushroom Salad with Gorgonzola, Peppers, and Bacon, 98
  Tamarind Pot Roast, 105
  Whole-Grain Rotini with Pork, Pumpkin, and Sage, 221
Portobello Mushroom Salad with Gorgonzola, Peppers, and Bacon, 98
Potatoes
  about: better brain functioning with, 83; nutritional benefits, 83
  Fondant Potatoes and Pearl Onions, 194
  Garlic Rosemary Mashed Potatoes, 227
  Homemade Scallion Hash Brown Cakes, 83
  Shepherd's Pie, 223
  Vegetable Stew with Cornmeal Dumplings, 142
Pot stickers, shrimp shiitake, 233
Poultry. See also Poultry, dinner recipes

about: best ways to cook, 87; ground turkey, 88; turkey breast, 223
Baked Ravioli, 158
Buffalo Chicken Macaroni and Cheese, 165
Chicken Nachos, 93
Chicken Ramen Soup, 179
Chicken Rub, 189
Chicken Seasoning, 185
Farfalle with Chicken and Pesto, 158
High-Protein Spaghetti, 164
Homemade Buffalo Wing Sauce, 188
Lemon-Herb Grilled Chicken Salad, 95
Low-Fat Chicken Bacon Ranch Sandwich, 89
Power Wrap, 72
Protein Scramble Bowl, 75
Pulled Chicken BBQ Sandwich, 93
Slow-Cooked Chicken, 87
Southwestern Fajitas, 90
Tricolor Penne, 166
Turkey Burgers, 88
Poultry, dinner recipes
about: turkey breast, 223
Baked Buffalo Chicken Strips, 102
Beer Can Chicken, 111
Chicken and Bean Burrito, 104
Chicken and Broccoli Fettuccine, 162
Lean Turkey Meatloaf, 113
Marinated Grilled Turkey Cutlets, 114
Mustard Pecan Chicken, 106
Pesto Pork Chops, 107
Shepherd's Pie, 223
Spice-Rubbed Roasted Turkey Breast, 218
Sun-Dried Tomato Stuffed Chicken, 103
Tuscan Chicken, 110
Pound Cake Minis, 238

Power Wrap, 72
Pressure Cooker Beef Bourguignon, 219
Pressure cookers, about, 219
Processed, sugary foods, eating, 270
Protein bars, 82
Protein Cheesecake, 251
Protein Guacamole, 213
Protein Piña Colada, 244
Protein powder, about, 240
Protein powder, smoothies with. See Drinks
Proteins
amino acids and, 17
balancing other macronutrients with, 15
beverages/smoothies with. See Drinks
for breakfast. See Breakfast
calculating daily needs, 38–39, 40
calorie values and, 14–15
complete, 17
functions of, 15
good and bad nutrient combos, 43
high-carb-day sources, 21
as macronutrients, 14
snacks with. See Snacks
sources of, 17, 18, 267
sweets with. See Desserts
Protein Scramble Bowl, 75
Protein Sludge, 215
Pudding, chocolate, 255
Pulled Chicken BBQ Sandwich, 93
Pumpkin
Pumpkin Pie Protein Shake, 246
Pumpkin Soup Base, 172
Whole-Grain Rotini with Pork, Pumpkin, and Sage, 221

Questions, frequently asked, 269–71
Quinoa
about: protein from, 17, 130
Lemon Quinoa, 133

Quinoa Burritos, 130
Quinoa with Mixed Vegetables, 202

Radishes, roasted Brussels sprouts and, 224
Rainbow chard, farro with Raspberries, 77
Ravioli, baked, 158
RDA, defined, 196
Recipes. See also Ingredients; specific main ingredients
measurement conversions, 275
reading and preparing, 42, 67
structuring meals using. See Meal plans
Red Beans and Rice, 143
Red Onion and Olive Focaccia, 153
Red peppers. See Peppers
Resources, additional, 273
Restaurants, eating at, 42
Reverse dieting, 61–63
Rice and wild rice
about: brown rice, 145; types of, 94; wild rice, 94, 232
Butternut Squash Rice, 193
Healthy Fried Rice, 94
Mini Vegetable Burgers, 145
Red Beans and Rice, 143
Rosemary Wild Rice Pilaf, 232
Summer Squash Casserole, 205
Ultimate Spinach and Mushroom Risotto, 201
Roasted Radishes and Brussels Sprouts, 224
Roasted Root Vegetables with Orange and Thyme, 230
Root vegetables. See also Carrots; Potatoes; Sweet potatoes
about, 148
Roasted Root Vegetables with Orange and Thyme, 230
Root Vegetable Salad, 148
Vegetable Stew with Cornmeal Dumplings, 142
Rosemary, about, 227
Rosemary Wild Rice Pilaf, 232

Rubs. *See* Sauces, dressings, and rubs
Rutabagas, 142, 148

Saag Tofu, 152
Sage-Parmesan Polenta, 199
Salads
    Apple Coleslaw, 147
    Arugula and Fennel Salad with Pomegranate, 146
    Asparagus Salad with Hard-Boiled Egg, 99
    Bean Salad with Orange Vinaigrette, 136
    Feta and Tuna Pasta Salad, 123
    Fresh Corn, Pepper, and Avocado Salad, 134
    Fruit Salad, 258
    Kale and Sea Vegetables with Orange-Sesame Dressing, 149
    Lemon-Herb Grilled Chicken Salad, 95
    Lentil Salad, 97
    Red Pepper and Fennel Salad, 150
    Root Vegetable Salad, 148
    Shrimp Orzo Salad, 163
    Simple Autumn Salad, 137
    Sirloin Chopped Salad, 90
    Southwestern Beet Slaw, 135
    Spicy Peanut Tempeh Salad, 131
    Tuna Salad, 92
Salmon. *See Fish and shellfish references*
Sandwiches and wraps
    about: best bread for, 89
    Chicken and Bean Burrito, 104
    High-Protein Tuna Melt, 124
    Low-Fat Chicken Bacon Ranch Sandwich, 89
    Mini Vegetable Burgers, 145
    Portobello Mushroom Salad with Gorgonzola, Peppers, and Bacon, 98
    Portobello Tacos, 139
    Power Wrap, 72

Pulled Chicken BBQ Sandwich, 93
Quinoa Burritos, 130
Salmon Burgers, 120
Spinach, Feta, and Pesto Chicken Quesadillas, 91
Steakhouse Blue Cheese Burger, 109
Turkey Burgers, 88
Vegetarian Cakes, 128
Sauces, dressings, and rubs, **181**–89
    about: making homemade seasonings, 184; making pesto, 91
    Adobo Seasoning, 184
    Balsamic Vinaigrette, 182
    Basil Pesto, 187
    Cajun Seasoning, 185
    Chicken Rub, 189
    Chicken Seasoning, 185
    Citrus Vinaigrette, 183
    Curry Seasoning, 186
    Dry Rub for Ribs, 189
    Easy Dumpling Dipping Sauce, 233
    French Dressing, 97
    Fresh Salsa, 80
    Homemade Buffalo Wing Sauce, 188
    Marinara Sauce, 112
    Orange-Sesame Dressing, 149
    Oriental Seasoning, 187
    Spicy Memphis Seasoning, 186
    Sun-Dried Tomato Vinaigrette, 183
    Vanilla Pear Vinaigrette, 184
Sausage
    about: types of, 96
    Protein Scramble Bowl, 75
    Sausage and Spicy Eggs, 96
Seafood. *See Fish and shellfish references*
Seasonings. *See* Sauces, dressings, and rubs
Sea vegetables, kale and, 149
Shallots, using, 192

Shepherd's Pie, 223
Shrimp. *See Fish and shellfish references*
    Shrimp Noodles with Chinese Chives, 167
Side dishes, **191**–205. *See also* Pasta; Salads
    Baked Eggplant and Bell Pepper, 131
    Broccoli-Cauliflower Bake, 203
    Butternut Squash Rice, 193
    Farro with Rainbow Chard, 198
    Fondant Potatoes and Pearl Onions, 194
    Garlicky Chickpeas and Spinach, 156
    Garlic Rosemary Mashed Potatoes, 227
    High-Protein Spread, 128
    Kohlrabi and Swiss Chard, 192
    Lemon Quinoa, 133
    Mushroom Barley Pilaf with Fresh Green Beans, 229
    Oyster Portobello Un-Stuffing, 226
    Pickled Asparagus, 197
    Quinoa with Mixed Vegetables, 202
    Red Beans and Rice, 143
    Roasted Beet Celeriac Mash, 195
    Roasted Radishes and Brussels Sprouts, 224
    Roasted Root Vegetables with Orange and Thyme, 230
    Rosemary Wild Rice Pilaf, 232
    Sage-Parmesan Polenta, 199
    Shrimp Shiitake Pot Stickers, 233
    Southwestern Beet Slaw, 135
    Spicy Roasted Spaghetti Squash, 196
    Stuffed Mushrooms, 204
    Summer Squash Casserole, 205
    Sweet and Spicy Brussels Sprouts, 155
    Ultimate Spinach and Mushroom Risotto, 201
    Whipped Butternut Squash, 228

Whipped Sweet Potatoes, 228
Zucchini Boats, 200
Zucchini Oven Fries, 132
Simple Autumn Salad, 137
Simple Sweet Potato Pancakes, 81
Sirloin Chopped Salad, 90
Slow-Cooked Chicken, 87
Slow Cooker Beef Stew, 178
Smoothies. *See* Drinks
Snacks, **207**–16
    Banana Protein Pudding, 209
    Chocolate-Covered Berry
      Delight, 214
    Cinnamon Apple Snack Bars, 211
    Cinnamon Protein Apple
      Slices, 212
    Garlic Kale Chips, 216
    Goat Cheese–Stuffed Dates,
      234
    Hard-Boiled Eggs, 212
    Herb Mashed Eggs, 213
    Mocha Protein Bars, 209
    No-Bake Apple Crisp, 208
    Nutty Cottage Cheese, 211
    Protein Guacamole, 213
    Protein Sludge, 215
    Southwestern Eggs, 214
    Sweet and Spicy Almonds, 235
    Triple Berry Parfait, 210
Soups and stews, **169**–80
    Black Bean and King Oyster
      Mushroom Soup, 177
    Butternut Squash and Apple Fall
      Soup, 177
    Cashew-Zucchini Soup, 151
    Chicken Ramen Soup, 179
    Corn and Black Bean Chili, 170
    Cream of Broccoli Soup, 180
    Creamy Cauliflower Soup, 176
    Creamy Corn Chowder, 171
    Pumpkin Soup Base, 172
    Slow Cooker Beef Stew, 178
    Spring Pea and Mint Soup, 175
    Sweet and Spicy Carrot
      Soup, 174
    Sweet Green Chickpea Soup, 175
    Sweet Potato Soup, 173

Vegetable Stew with Cornmeal
    Dumplings, 142
    Southwestern Beet Slaw, 135
Southwestern Eggs, 214
Southwestern Fajitas, 90
Southwestern Omelet, 71
Spaghetti, high-protein, 164
Spaghetti Marinara with Chicken
    and Basil, 112
Spaghetti squash. *See* Squash
Spice-Rubbed Roasted Turkey
    Breast, 218
Spices. *See* Herbs and spices
Spicy Peanut Tempeh Salad, 131
Spicy Roasted Spaghetti
    Squash, 196
Spinach
    about: nutritional/bone
      benefits, 79
    Garlicky Chickpeas and
      Spinach, 156
    Greek Egg Scramble, 70
    Saag Tofu, 152
    Spinach, Feta, and Pesto
      Chicken Quesadillas, 91
    Spinach, Red Onion, and
      Mushroom Frittata, 79
    Spinach and Feta Salmon, 119
    Super Greens Shake, 247
    Ultimate Spinach and Mushroom
      Risotto, 201
    Vegetable-Stuffed Poblano
      Peppers, 138
Spring Pea and Mint Soup, 175
Squash
    about: versatility of, 205
    Butternut Squash and Apple Fall
      Soup, 177
    Butternut Squash Rice, 193
    Cashew-Zucchini Soup, 151
    Spaghetti Squash Crab Blend,
      89
    Spicy Roasted Spaghetti
      Squash, 196
    Summer Squash Casserole, 205
    Summer Vegetable Tian, 154
    Vegetable Baked Ziti, 225

    Vegetable-Stuffed Poblano
      Peppers, 138
    Whipped Butternut Squash, 228
    Zucchini Boats, 200
    Zucchini Oven Fries, 132
Steakhouse Blue Cheese
    Burger, 109
Strawberries. *See* Berries
Strength training. *See* Exercise
Stuffed Mushrooms, 204
Stuffed Salmon Fillets, 121
Stuffing, oyster portobello
    un-stuffing, 226
Sugary foods, eating, 270
Summer Squash Casserole, 205
Summer Vegetable Tian, 154
Sun-dried tomatoes. *See* Tomatoes
Super Greens Shake, 247
Supplements, 270
Sweet and Spicy Almonds, 235
Sweet and Spicy Brussels
    Sprouts, 155
    Sweet Green Chickpea Soup, 175
Sweet potatoes
    Roasted Root Vegetables with
      Orange and Thyme, 230
    Simple Sweet Potato
      Pancakes, 81
    Sweet Potato Soup, 173
    Whipped Sweet Potatoes, 228
Swiss chard, kohlrabi and, 192

Tacos, portobello, 139
    Tamarind Pot Roast, 105
Tea. *See* Drinks
Tempeh salad, spicy peanut, 131
Thyme, about, 230
Tians, 154
Tilapia, 123, 124
Tiramisu Smoothie, 245
Tofu
    about: types of, 152
    High-Protein Spread, 128
    Saag Tofu, 152
Tomatoes
    Fresh Salsa, 80
    Marinara Sauce, 112

Tomatoes—*continued*
    Summer Vegetable Tian, 154
    Sun-Dried Tomato Stuffed
      Chicken, 103
    Sun-Dried Tomato Tuna, 121
    Sun-Dried Tomato
      Vinaigrette, 183
    Vegetable-Stuffed Poblano
      Peppers, 138
Tortillas
    Chicken and Bean Burrito,
      104
    Chicken Nachos, 93
    Huevos Rancheros, 80
    Portobello Tacos, 139
    Quinoa Burritos, 130
    Spinach, Feta, and Pesto
      Chicken Quesadillas, 91
Training. *See* Exercise
Tricolor Penne, 166
Triple Berry Parfait, 210
Tropical Blend Smoothie, 246
Tuna. *See Fish and shellfish
references*
Turkey. *See Poultry references*
Turkey bacon. *See* Bacon
Turnips, 142, 148
Tuscan Chicken, 110
Two-Minute Chocolate Strawberry
    Protein Bowl, 75

Ultimate Spinach and Mushroom
    Risotto, 201

Vanilla
    Neapolitan Smoothie, 241
    Vanilla-Peach Dessert Bars, 256
    Vanilla Pear Vinaigrette, 184
    Vanilla Raspberry Protein
      Fluff, 77
Vegan mains, sides, and
    salads, **141**–56
    about: cashew nut butter, 151
    Apple Coleslaw, 147
    Arugula and Fennel Salad with
      Pomegranate, 146
    Cashew-Zucchini Soup, 151

    Garlicky Chickpeas and
      Spinach, 156
    Kale and Sea Vegetables with
      Orange-Sesame Dressing, 149
    Mediterranean Chickpea
      Bake, 144
    Mini Vegetable Burgers, 145
    Red Beans and Rice, 143
    Red Onion and Olive
      Focaccia, 153
    Red Pepper and Fennel
      Salad, 150
    Root Vegetable Salad, 148
    Saag Tofu, 152
    Summer Vegetable Tian, 154
    Sweet and Spicy Brussels
      Sprouts, 155
    Vegetable Stew with Cornmeal
      Dumplings, 142
Vegetables. *See also specific
vegetables*
about: adding green veggies
    to all meals, 45; blood
    sugar and, 28; canning, 197;
    nutritional benefits, 28
    Healthy Fried Rice, 94
    Protein Scramble Bowl, 75
    Quinoa with Mixed
      Vegetables, 202
    Southwestern Beet Slaw, 135
    Vegetable Baked Ziti, 225
    Vegetable-Stuffed Poblano
      Peppers, 138
Vegetarian mains, sides, and
    salads, **127**–39
    Baked Eggplant and Bell
      Pepper, 131
    Banana Oatmeal, 129
    Bean Salad with Orange
      Vinaigrette, 136
    Fresh Corn, Pepper, and
      Avocado Salad, 134
    High-Protein Spread, 128
    Lemon Quinoa, 133
    Portobello Tacos, 139
    Quinoa Burritos, 130
    Simple Autumn Salad, 137

    Southwestern Beet Slaw, 135
    Spicy Peanut Tempeh Salad, 131
    Vegetable-Stuffed Poblano
      Peppers, 138
    Vegetarian Cakes, 128
    Zucchini Oven Fries, 132
Vinaigrette. *See* Sauces, dressings,
    and rubs

Walnut oil, 150
Water intake, 45
Weekly depletion and
    re-feed, 56–57
Whipped Butternut Squash, 228
Whipped Sweet Potatoes, 228
Whole-Grain Rotini with Pork,
    Pumpkin, and Sage, 221
Whole-Wheat Penne with Kale and
    Cannellini Beans, 159
Wild rice pilaf, 232
Working out. *See* Exercise

Yogurt
    about: best Greek yogurt, 75
    Banana Protein Pudding, 209
    Berries and Cream Parfait, 78
    Blue Velvet Smoothie, 241
    Chocolate-Covered Berry
      Delight, 214
    Cinnamon-Pear Frozen
      Yogurt, 257
    Mixed Berry Frozen Yogurt, 255
    Orange Cream Delight, 243
    Peaches and Cream
      Smoothie, 243
    Peanut Butter and Jelly
      Smoothie, 244
    Peanut Butter Banana Frozen
      Greek Yogurt, 251
    Simple Sweet Potato
      Pancakes, 81
    Triple Berry Parfait, 210
    Two-Minute Chocolate
      Strawberry Protein Bowl, 75

Zucchini. *See* Squash